DOCTORS'
HOME
REMEDIES

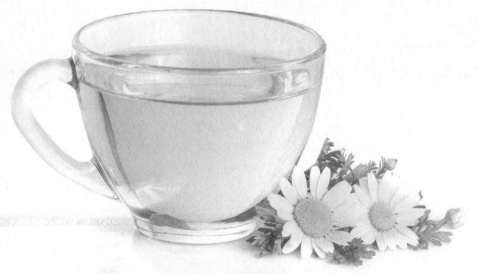

Publications International, Ltd.

Table of Contents

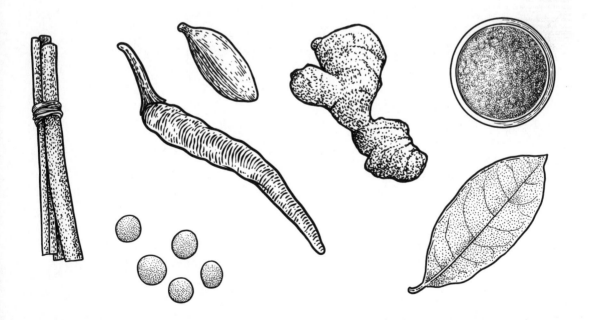

How Can Home Remedies Help?

Do you sometimes wish you had a doctor in the family? A pro in the know with answers to your medical questions, both mundane and life threatening. With *Doctors' Home Remedies*, we present the next best thing. Plus, you won't have to deal with the hassle of scheduling an appointment, sitting in the waiting room, or spending money on yet another copay.

These days, we're bombarded by advertisements for prescription and over-the-counter medications. There's a drug for every symptom and every condition—and then some! The constant promotion would have you believe that medications are our only treatment options.

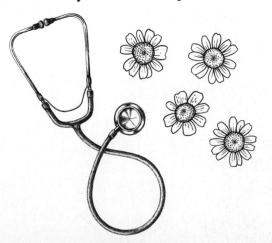

But there are simple solutions to everyday problems, using common products that are sitting on your shelves, in your cabinets, and even in your refrigerator. Many of these are time-tested remedies; however, others are more recent discoveries, based on the latest scientific information.

With *Doctors' Home Remedies* we provide you with a wealth of knowledge to help you solve many day-to-day illnesses and conditions. Chapter 1 delves into "Food Cures," emphasizing some of the most essential foods for good health. You will learn about the power of these foods and the importance of a healthy diet. Chapter 2 focuses on "Apple Cider Vinegar," and provides home remedies that have been cherished for centuries. In addition to the benefits of apple cider vinegar, Chapter 2 goes in depth on the many other varieties of vinegar that can also improve your life. Chapter 3 explores how to "Soothe Everyday Aches & Pains" using natural remedies to heal arthritis, headaches, sprains, and strains. For instance, did you know that celery and celery seeds can act as an anti-inflammatory alleviating pain during acute arthritis attacks? Chapter 4 is called "Nature's Antibiotics." This chapter primarily provides home remedies for digestive problems, sore throats, congestion, colds, and the flu. Chapter 5 has more of a beauty-centric theme as it suggests how to achieve "Healthy Skin, Hair, & Nails" naturally. And finally, Chapter 6 is entitled "More Remedies & Cures." This chapter is a collection of doctor-approved remedies for common conditions for men and women of all ages.

We hope you find this book insightful and helpful, and most importantly, a source you can rely on for simple solutions to get well and stay well.

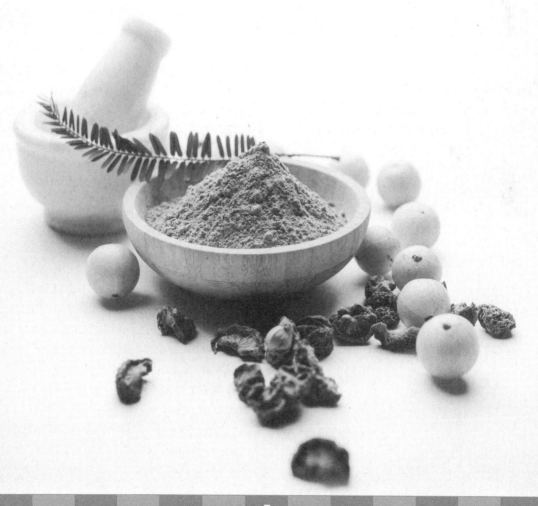

Chapter 1: Food Cures

How Does My Diet Affect Me?

Many of the most common health problems we face today—from annoying problems like constipation to more serious conditions such as heart disease—are linked to what we eat. Within the last several decades, the focus of research into possible links between nutrition and health has expanded; it now includes not only the potential dangers of eating certain foods (or too much of certain foods) but also the natural healing and protective powers that some foods possess.

That's not to say that food alone can cure disease or take the place of medical treatment. It is, however, becoming increasingly evident that food has disease-fighting potential. Translation? You have the power to choose foods that may help prevent and treat a host of today's most common maladies.

The more we research, the more proof we have: Eating well and good health are intertwined. Eating right can't prevent or cure every illness—but eating nutrient-dense foods that give us the vitamins and minerals we need is necessary for good long-term health. More than that, for a number of chronic conditions, including certain foods in your diet—or excluding others—can help soothe symptoms, forestall further health problems, and even reverse the progression of the disease.

The Best Diet?

We often wonder what to eat to maintain optimum health. To some extent the answers are personal. Bodies are different, and the best diet for you will be the one that gives you the most energy and makes you feel the best. However, we do know some general guidelines for eating for good health:

🍃 Eat meals heavy on vegetables, fruits, and grains.

🍴 Eat an array of vegetables, in all colors. For leafy green vegetables, the darker the green, the more nutrients are available.

🍴 Eat red meat sparingly.

🍴 Eat fish a few times each week. Fatty fish like salmon and tuna carry an array of health benefits.

🍴 Every so often, we hear about a new "superfood." Many are overhyped—no single food is a miracle food—but yogurt, berries, salmon, dark leafy greens, and beans and other legumes are all packed with nutrients and offer a variety of health benefits.

The Role of Multivitamins

Getting enough of essential nutrients is a good start on the road to a healthy immune system. And generally, eating a well-balanced diet will get you on that road. But you may be thinking about taking a multivitamin to help fill in the gaps. Are they worth it? And what should you look for? Most nutrition experts would tell you to get the majority of your nutrients from food—mostly because there are other good-for-you components in food that a specific vitamin may not offer. Taking a multivitamin is a good backup plan. If you decide to take a multivitamin, follow these tips:

🍴 Look for a vitamin/mineral combination. You need vitamins and minerals to enhance your immune system, so be sure the product you choose has all you need.

🍴 Don't use products that have more than 100 percent of the recommended daily allowance (RDA) or daily value (DV) of a nutrient. You're going to get most of your vitamins and minerals from your diet, so don't go overboard.

🍴 Make sure your multivitamin meets your needs. If you need to boost your immune system, look for a multivitamin that has vitamin E, C, B6, and zinc.

🍴 Check the expiration date. Multivitamins may not start smelling up the place after they expire, but they can lose their potency.

🍴 Only take what is recommended. One a day is exactly what you should take. Don't double up on pills.

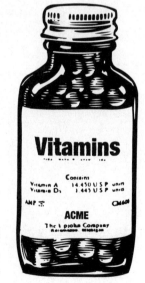

Essential Foods for Health

When it comes to putting healing medicine in an easy-to-swallow package, Mother Nature has truly outdone science. Fortunately, science is catching on and gradually uncovering the many ways that food, especially food in its natural state, appears able to help the body heal and protect itself. With the aid of this chapter, you can put that newly discovered knowledge to work for your own health's sake, with each food you choose and each bite you take.

Apricots

Apricots are chock-full of beta-carotene and other carotenoids, the beautiful pigments that color fruits and vegetables. There are more than 400 different kinds and most, if not all, are antioxidants. Some of apricots' carotenoids such as lycopene, gamma carotene, and cryptoxanthin pack a much more powerful antioxidant punch than does beta-carotene, making them even more useful as cancer-fighters.

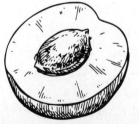

Apricots contain some vitamin C, which keeps skin and tissues supple and healthy. Vitamin C also has antioxidant properties and supports the immune system, helping the body make substances to fight off illnesses. Apricots are rich in fiber for their size, especially soluble fiber. This heart-healthy fiber lowers blood cholesterol levels and helps people with diabetes maintain stable blood sugar levels. You can count on apricots' insoluble fiber to keep the colon free of toxins and your bowels moving regularly.

Dried apricots, because they are concentrated, are a good source of iron. Three and a half ounces provide about 47 percent of the recommended dietary allowance for men and 31 percent for women.

Beets and Beet Greens

Beets have long been valued for their rich flavor, sweet taste, and vital nutrients. Beets are particularly rich in the B vitamin folate, which is essential for preventing a certain type of anemia and birth defects that affect the spinal column. Folate may prevent cancer, too, by protecting the DNA in cells from damage and mutation. Mutated cells are

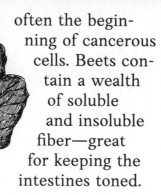

often the beginning of cancerous cells. Beets contain a wealth of soluble and insoluble fiber—great for keeping the intestines toned.

Beet greens are packed with healing nutrients, including disease fighters such as vitamin A and potassium. Calcium, too, is available from this nutritional powerhouse. The variety of vitamins and minerals make these leafy greens an all-around heart-healthy vegetable. If you are trying to quit smoking, beet greens may become your new friend. Just like soil, human blood has a pH value, and a slightly alkaline condition apparently triggers nicotine to stay in the blood longer, reducing the craving for more cigarettes. At the University of Nebraska Medical Center, researchers found that beet greens push blood pH slightly toward the alkaline side. Smokers who are trying to quit might try eating plenty of alkaline foods to reduce their need for nicotine. Other high-alkaline foods include dandelion greens, spinach, and raisins.

Beet greens are abundant in folate. This B vitamin protects lung cells from damage that can trigger cancer, so smokers get a double dose of prevention from these greens.

Cabbage

Cabbage juice has been used to prevent and heal ulcers for more than 40 years. Current research at the Stanford University School of Medicine revealed that when ulcer patients drank 1 quart of raw cabbage juice each day, ulcers in the stomach and small intestine healed in about five days. People who ate cabbage instead of drinking the juice also had faster healing times than those who did not eat cabbage.

Cabbage accomplishes this by killing bacteria, including the ulcer-causing *H. pylori*. Secondly, it contains a phytochemical called gefarnate that coaxes stomach cells into making extra mucus, which protects the stomach wall from digestive acid. As a cruciferous family member, cabbages of all types help fight the war on cancer. Two types of darker-colored war on cancer. Two types of darker-colored savoy cabbage and bok choy—also provide beta-carotene.

Carrots

Modern science has determined that carrots do much more than help eyesight. They offer a natural defense against heart disease, strokes, cancer, cataracts, and even constipation. And it only takes one carrot a day to dramatically reduce health risks. Studies show that a humble carrot a day reduced the risk of heart attack in women by 22 percent, and a carrot a day five days per week reduced women's stroke risk by 68 percent. Women who did have a stroke were less likely to die or be disabled. Scientists believe that phytochemicals (plant chemicals) in carrots protect oxygen-deprived brain cells.

Lung cancer risk plunged by 60 percent in a different study when a carrot was eaten twice a week. The incidence of other cancers, such as stomach, mouth, and those of the female reproductive tract, are also decreased by eating carrots.

One raw carrot or 1/2 cup cooked carrots supplies two to three times the recommended daily intake of vitamin A in the form of protective beta-carotene. Carrots contain other carotenoids that are even more potent cancer warriors than beta-carotene: alpha-carotene, gamma-carotene, lycopene, and lutein.

Fennel

This familiar culinary herb is considered a digestive aid and a carminative, or agent capable of diminishing gas in the intestines. It is recommended for numerous complaints related to excessive gas in the stomach and intestines, including indigestion, cramps, and bloating, as well as for colic in infants. Other Umbelliferae family members such as dill and caraway are also considered carminatives.

As an antispasmodic, fennel acts on the smooth muscle of the respiratory passages as well as the stomach and intestines, which is the reason that fennel preparations are used to relieve bronchial spasms. Since it relaxes bronchial passages, allowing them to open wider, it is sometimes included in asthma, bronchitis, and cough formulas.

Fennel is also known to have an estrogenic effect and has long been used to promote milk production in nursing mothers.

Garlic

The tiny garlic clove may play a big role in lowering cholesterol, reducing the risk of heart disease, heart attacks, and stroke. Garlic contains several powerful antioxidants—compounds that prevent oxidation, a harmful process in the body. One of them is selenium, a mineral that is a component of glutathione peroxidase, a powerful antioxidant that the body makes to defend itself. Glutathione peroxidase works with vitamin E to form a super antioxidant defense system.

Other antioxidants in garlic include vitamin C, which helps reduce the damage that LDL cholesterol can cause, and quercetin, a phytochemical. (Phytochemicals are chemical substances found in plants that may have health benefits for people.) Garlic also has trace amounts of the mineral manganese, which is an important component of an antioxidant enzyme called superoxide dismutase.

Arteries benefit greatly from the protection antioxidants provide. And garlic's ability to stop the oxidation of cholesterol may be one of the many ways it protects heart health. Garlic also appears to help prevent calcium from binding with other substances that lodge themselves in plaque. In a UCLA Medical Center study, 19 people were given either a placebo or an aged garlic extract that contained S-allylcysteine, one of garlic's sulfur-rich compounds, for one year. The placebo group had a significantly greater increase in their calcium score (22.2 percent) than the group that received the aged garlic extract (calcium score of 7.5 percent). The results of this small pilot study suggest that aged garlic extract may inhibit the rate of coronary artery calcification.

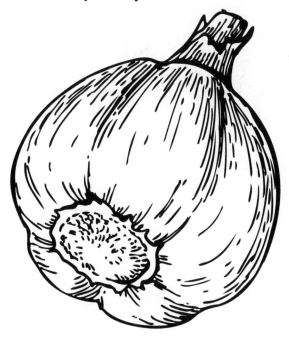

Research suggests that garlic can help make small improvements in blood pressure by increasing the blood flow to the capillaries, which are the tiniest blood vessels. The chemicals in garlic achieve this by causing the capillary walls to open wider and reducing the ability of blood platelets to stick together and cause blockages. Reductions are small—10 mmHg (millimeters of mercury, the unit of measurement for blood pressure) or less. This means if your blood pressure is 130 over 90 mmHg, garlic might help lower it to 120 over 80 mmHg. That's a slight improvement, but, along with some simple lifestyle adjustments, such as getting more exercise, garlic might help move your blood pressure out of the danger zone.

Horseradish

Have you ever bitten into a roast beef sandwich and thought your nose was on fire? The sandwich probably contained horseradish. Even a tiny taste of this potent condiment seems to go straight to your nose. Whether on a sandwich or in a herbal preparation, horseradish clears sinuses, increases facial circulation, and promotes expulsion of mucus.

Horseradish is helpful for sinus infections because it encourages your body to get rid of mucus. One way a sinus infection starts is with the accumulation of thick mucus in the sinuses: Stagnant mucus is the perfect breeding ground for bacteria to multiply and cause a painful infection. Horseradish can help thin and move out older, thicker mucus accumulations. If you are prone to developing sinus infections, try taking horseradish the minute you feel a cold coming on. Herbalists also recommend horseradish for common colds, influenza, and lung congestion. Incidentally, don't view the increase of mucus production after horseradish therapy as a sign your cold is worsening. The free-flowing mucus is a positive sign that your body is ridding itself of wastes. Horseradish has a mild natural antibiotic effect and it stimulates production. Thus, it has been used for urinary infections.

Mint

Mint is one of the most reliable home remedies for an upset stomach. Grandmas throughout the world have been handing out mints for centuries to treat indigestion, flatulence, and colic. The two types of mint you're most likely to encounter are spearmint and peppermint. Although they once were considered the same plant, peppermint actually is a natural hybrid of spearmint. It's also the more potent of the herbs. Use peppermint leaves to brew soothing teas.

Peppermint owes part of its healing power to an aromatic oil called menthol. Spearmint's primary active constituent is a similar but weaker chemical called carvone. Oil of peppermint contains up to 78 percent menthol. Menthol encourages bile (a fluid secreted by the liver) to flow into the duodenum, where it promotes digestion. Menthol is also a potent antispasmodic; in other words, it calms the action of muscles, particularly those of the digestive system.

Melons

Melons come in a wide variety of shapes, sizes, and flavors, yet have certain healing nutrients in common. Their high levels of potassium benefit the heart. Some melons have health-boosting phytochemicals and top-notch amounts of vitamins C and A. Orange-fleshed melons, such as cantaloupe, are high in beta-carotene. One cup of melon cubes supplies nearly everyone's daily requirement for vitamin A. When studying endometrial cancer, researchers at the University of Alabama reported that women who did not have this cancer had eaten at least one food high in beta-carotene, such as cantaloupe, every day. The women who had endometrial cancer had eaten less than one beta-carotene food per week.

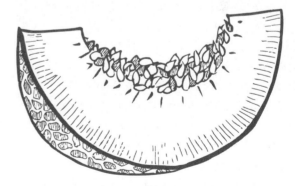

The red pulp from watermelons is teeming with a different carotenoid, lycopene. Lycopene is even more potent than beta-carotene at doing away with free radicals, those damaging molecules that can be the culprits in heart disease, cancer, and cataracts. High intakes of lycopene, though not watermelon itself as yet, are linked to a decreased incidence of prostate cancer.

Oats

You might think oatmeal is the most boring bowl of breakfast food around, but oats are a fantastic source of healing nourishment. They contain starches, proteins, vitamins, and minerals, and though they contain some fat, they are low in saturated fat, which makes them a healthy choice. A serving of hot oat bran cereal provides about 4 grams of dietary fiber (health professionals recommend we consume 20 to 35 grams of fiber each day). Some types of dietary fiber bind to cholesterol, and since this form of fiber is not absorbed by the body, neither is the cholesterol. A number of clinical trials have found that regular consumption of oat bran reduces blood cholesterol levels in just one month. High fiber diets may also reduce the risk of colon and rectal cancer.

Oats have been used topically to heal wounds and various skin rashes and diseases. The familiar sticky-but-smooth consistency of cooked oats is emulated in many oat products; as a result they have muci-laginous, demulcent, and soothing qualities. Soaps and various bath and body products made from oats are readily available. Oatmeal baths are wonderful for soothing dry, flaky skin or allaying itching in cases of poison oak and chicken pox.

Because oats are believed to have a calming effect, herbalists recommend them to help ease the frustration and anxiety that often accompany nicotine and drug withdrawal. Oats contain the alkaloid gramine, which has been credited with mild sedative properties. Scientists have conducted clinical trials to determine whether oats may help treat drug addiction or reduce nicotine craving, but the evidence is inconclusive.

Olive Oil

A diet that is rich in olive oil has enhanced the health of people living in the Mediterranean region for thousands of years. Within the past century, however, olive oil's benefits have also been scientifically investigated, acknowledged, and proclaimed across the globe.

There are two important polyunsaturated fats that are essential for human health, but the body cannot make them. This means we must get them from the foods we eat. These two essential fatty acids are alpha-linolenic acid, an omega-3 fatty acid, and linoleic acid, an omega-6 fatty acid. The body gets both from olive oil. Omega-3 oils are the healthiest. They are part of a group of substances called prostaglandins that help keep blood cells from sticking together, increase blood flow, and reduce inflammation. This makes omega-3 oils useful in preventing cardiovascular disease as well as inflammatory conditions, such as arthritis.

Omega-6 oils are healthy, too, but they are not quite as helpful as omega-3's. Omega-6's can help form prostaglandins that are similarly beneficial to the ones produced by omega 3's, but they can also produce harmful prostaglandins. The unfavorable prostaglandins increase blood-cell stickiness and promote cardiovascular disease, and they also appear to be linked to the formation of cancer. To encourage your body to make beneficial prostaglandins from omega-6 oils, you should decrease the amount of animal fats you eat. Too many animal fats tend to push your body into using omega-6 oils to make the unfavorable prostaglandins rather than the helpful ones.

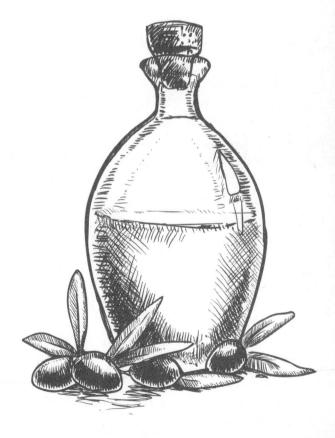

The research is inconclusive about how much omega-6 you should eat compared to the amount of omega-3. Many researchers suggest consuming one to four times more omega-6's than omega-3's. However, the typical American eats anywhere from 11 to 30 times more omega-6's than omega-3's. The U.S. Dietary Reference Intakes for essential fatty acids recommends the consumption of omega-6 and omega-3 fats in a ratio of 10-to-1. This means consuming ten times more omega-6's than omega-3's. Lucky for us, nature provided that exact ratio of fat in each little olive. The linoleic-to-linolenic ratio is about 10-to-1.

Soy

When you think soy, you probably think tofu. But there's more to soy—and it's worth considering. The evidence linking soy protein and heart-disease prevention was so compelling that the Food and Drug Administration approved a health claim for use on food labels stating: "25 grams of soy protein per day, as part of a diet low in saturated fat and cholesterol, may reduce the risk of heart disease."

For many, getting this much soy in the diet is a challenge. Fortunately, soy foods are more widely available these days, and more versatile, so the choices extend far beyond the traditional tofu and soy milk. For instance, a simple substitution of soy flour for up to 30 percent of all-purpose flour is an easy way to sneak in soy. Soy protein isolate, a powdered form of soy, can be added to a smoothie, sprinkled over cereal, or mixed in a casserole dish. Even easier and especially good for the soy wary are the veggie burgers, energy bars, breakfast cereals, and snack foods made from soy commonly available today.

Spinach

Spinach's beautiful deep green color is a tip-off that it contains plenty of beta-carotene; those orange and red carotene pigments are hiding beneath the dark green chlorophyll. Spinach is also an excellent source of vitamin C, folate, and iron.

Spinach is a cornucopia of cancer fighters. For example, it has triple the amount of lutein and four times the amount of beta-carotene as broccoli. These antioxidants not only help prevent cancer, heart disease, and cataracts, but also boost the immune system. One study found that eating spinach more than twice a week was correlated with reduced risk of breast cancer. This vegetable contains a lot of folate, too. McGill University researchers found that folate improves serotonin levels in the brain, inducing a feeling of well-being. A daily dose of cooked spinach alleviated depression in study participants.

Spinach has the mineral manganese, too, which works with other minerals to strengthen bones. Although spinach is rich in calcium, the body is not able to absorb much of it. That's because spinach contains a compound called oxalic acid that binds with calcium, making it unavailable to the body. People who are prone to developing the most common type of kidney stones will want to limit their intake of spinach because the oxalic acid in this food can promote the formation of stones.

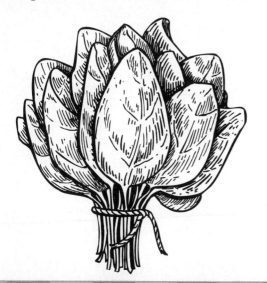

Sweet Potatoes

Sweet potatoes are among the unsung heroes of healthy eating. Nutrient-packed with only a few calories, sweet potatoes support immune function, eyesight, heart health, and cancer protection.

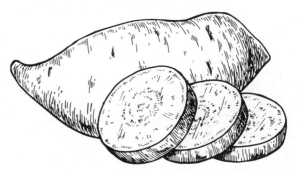

Teeming with beta-carotene, sweet potatoes outrank carrots by far in this healthful nutrient. This beneficial antioxidant wages a continuous battle against free radicals and the diseases they trigger, including cancer. In a study at Harvard University, people who ate one cup of cooked sweet potatoes, carrots, or spinach every day (all foods high in beta-carotene) had a 40 percent lower risk of experiencing a stroke. Researchers theorized that this nutrient protects blood cholesterol from undergoing damage from oxygen molecules. Damaged cholesterol begins the artery-clogging process. Other studies show that the more beta-carotene and vitamin A stroke patients have in their bloodstream, the less likely they are to die from the stroke and the more likely they are to make a full recovery.

All this beta-carotene also promotes healthy eyes and vision, since much of it gets turned into vitamin A as the body needs it. This wonder nutrient also works with certain white blood cells, tuning up your immune system to fight off colds, flu, and other illnesses. Sweet potatoes rank right up with bananas as a source of potassium, the heart-friendly nutrient. These colorful roots are a surprisingly good source of vitamin C.

Swiss Chard

This gently flavored vegetable is chock-full of beta-carotene and its relatives lutein and zeaxanthin, all potent disease fighters and immune boosters. The minerals potassium and magnesium, along with vitamin C, also hide in these beautifully colored, crinkled leaves.

Chard's carotenoids are strong protectors against cancer, heart disease, strokes, cataracts, and maybe even aging. Studies have not addressed whether eating chard confers these same protective benefits. Some researchers believe that

antioxidants such as these prevent wear and tear on cells, thus reducing the number of times they need to reproduce within a person's lifetime and possibly slowing down the aging process. Chard also contains reasonable amounts of vitamin C, another antioxidant.

Even though chard is full of calcium and iron, like spinach, it's not very absorbable. Chard, too, is rich in oxalic acid, which binds these minerals. Some people shy away from chard, having heard that it is high in sodium. One-half cup cooked chard does contain 158 mg of sodium, but this is just a fraction of the daily maximum recommended of 2400 mg. (However, our bodies only need 200 mg per day.) Processed foods such as crackers, chips, canned soups, and lunchmeats have many times more sodium than chard, and often without the plethora of healing nutrients.

Water

That's right—water. Every part of your body relies on water. Without it, you wouldn't live long—four or five days at the most. Your blood, for example, is more than three quarters water. Other body fluids, such as saliva and digestive juices, are primarily water, as is urine. You couldn't get rid of body wastes without it. Almost every chemical reaction in the body takes place in a water medium; water also lubricates and protects the joints, organs, nose, and mouth. Your body needs water so that when you get hot, you can sweat. The water you sweat off then evaporates on your skin, cooling you down.

So how much do you need to drink? Generally, you should drink six to eight cups of water a day. Although you can get by on less, drinking this much water is espe-

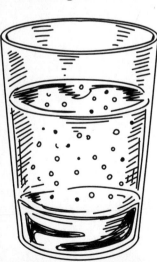

cially kind to your kidneys and colon because it helps flush toxins out of your body. When you drink a lot of water, the toxins can't hang around long enough to cause damage to your kidneys or cancerous growths in the colon. In fact, drinking plenty of water may be the simplest of all disease prevention tips.

Why not just drink when you're thirsty? Because your body's thirst-o-meter isn't very reliable. You should drink about three cups more than your thirst tells you to. And as you get older, your body loses the ability to tell when it's thirsty, making it doubly important to drink water even when you don't crave a cool drink.

Yogurt

Yogurt (along with some of its other fermented dairy cousins, like kefir) was a long-established staple in Eastern Europe and the Middle East before it reached our shores. And there was a time when yogurt eaters in this country were considered "health nuts." Our attitudes have changed considerably. Today, yogurt is commonly consumed by men, women, and children of all ages. Walk into any supermarket today, and you'll see that the varieties and flavors of this nutritious food take up considerable space in the dairy section.

Yogurt may not be the miracle food some have claimed, but it certainly has a lot to offer in the health department. Besides being an excellent source of bone-building calcium, it is believed that the bacterial cultures *Lactobacillus bulgaricus* and *Streptococcus thermophilus* that are used to make yogurt carry their own health benefits. For example, research has suggested that eating yogurt regularly helps boost the body's immune system function, warding off colds and possibly even helping to fend off cancer. It is also thought the friendly bacteria found in many types of yogurt can help prevent and even remedy diarrhea.

For people who suffer from lactose intolerance, yogurt is often well tolerated because live yogurt cultures produce lactase, making the lactose sugar in the yogurt easier to digest. Be sure to check the label on the yogurt carton for the National Yogurt Association's Live and Active Cultures (LAC) seal. This seal identifies products that contain a significant amount of live and active cultures. But don't look to frozen yogurt as an option; most frozen yogurt contains little of the healthful bacteria.

There is a dizzying array of brands and varieties of yogurts in most supermarkets. But there are some basic traits to look for when deciding which to put in your cart. Choose a yogurt that is either low fat or fat free. It should contain no more than three grams of fat per eight-ounce carton. Some yogurts are also sugar free (these are often signaled by the term "light," but check the label to be sure, since this term might also refer to fat content) and contain an alternative sweetener instead of added sugar. Consider choosing plain, vanilla, lemon, or any one of the yogurts without a fruit mixture added. The mixture adds calories and little if anything in the way of vitamins, minerals, or fiber. Your best health bet is to add your own fresh fruit to plain fat-free yogurt.

Yogurt must always be refrigerated. Each carton should have a "sell by" date stamped on it. It should be eaten within the week following the "sell by" date to take full advantage of the live and active cultures in the yogurt. As yogurt is stored, the amount of live and active cultures begins to decline.

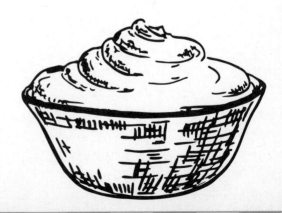

Chapter 2: Apple Cider Vinegar

What Exactly Is Vinegar?

Vinegar is a dilute solution of acetic acid that results from a two-step fermentation process. The first step is the fermentation of sugar into alcohol, usually by yeast. Any natural source of sugar can be used. For example, the sugar may be derived from the juice, or cider, of fruit (such as grapes, apples, raisins, or even coconuts); from a grain (such as barley or rice); from honey, molasses, or sugar cane; or even, in the case of certain distilled vinegars, from the cellulose in wood (such as beech).

What you have at the end of this first phase, then, is an alcohol-containing liquid, such as wine (from grapes), beer (from barley), hard cider (from apples), or another fermented liquid. The alcoholic liquid used to create a vinegar is generally reflected in the vinegar's name—for example, red wine vinegar, white wine vinegar, malt vinegar, or cider vinegar.

In the second phase of the vinegar-production process, certain naturally occurring bacteria known as acetobacters combine the alcohol-containing liquid with oxygen to form the acetic-acid solution we call vinegar. Acetic acid is what gives vinegar its sour taste. Although time-consuming, this second phase of the process will happen without human intervention if the alcoholic liquid is exposed to oxygen long enough.

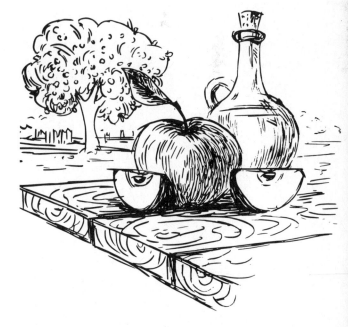

About Acidity

The U.S. Food and Drug Administration requires that vinegar contain a minimum of 4 percent acetic acid. White vinegar is typically 5 percent acetic acid, and cider and wine vinegars are a bit more acidic, usually between 5 percent and 6 percent. A little acidity goes a long way—acetic acid is in fact corrosive and can destroy living tissues when concentrated. An acetic acid level of 11 percent or more can burn the skin. And according to the Consumer Product Safety Commission, an "acetic acid preparation containing free or chemically unneutralized acetic acid in a concentration of 20 percent or more" is considered poison. In fact, a 20 percent acetic acid concentration is sometimes used as an herbicide to kill garden weeds.

A History of Vinegar

The first vinegar was the result of an ancient, serendipitous, accident. Once upon a time, a keg of wine (presumably a poorly sealed one that allowed oxygen in) was stored too long, and when the would-be drinkers opened it, they found a sour liquid instead of wine. The name "vinegar" is derived from the French words for "sour wine." Fortunately, our resourceful ancestors found ways to use the "bad" wine.

They put it to work as a cure-all, a food preservative, and later, a flavor enhancer. It wasn't long before they figured out how to make vinegar on purpose, and producing it became one of the world's earliest commercial industries.

Scientists believe wine originated during the Neolithic period (approximately 8500 B.C. to 4000 B.C., when humans first began farming and crafting stone tools) in Egypt and the Middle East. Large pottery jugs dating back to 6000 B.C. that were unearthed in archaeological digs possessed a strange yellow residue. Chemical analysis revealed the residue contained calcium tartrate, which is formed from tartaric acid, a substance that occurs naturally in large amounts only in grapes. So, the traces strongly suggest the jugs were used to make or hold wine.

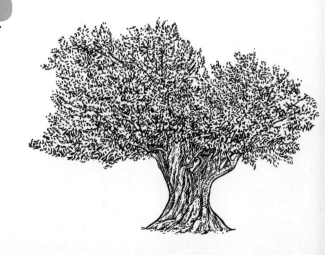

Considering the slow grape-pressing methods used at that time and the heat of the desert environment, grape juice would likely have fermented into wine quite quickly. Likewise, the wine would have turned to vinegar rapidly, if conditions were right. So how did these ancient people—who had only recently (in evolutionary terms) begun planting their own food and fashioning tools—manage to understand and control fermentation enough to prevent all their wine from turning to vinegar before they could drink it? Based on evidence found in archaeological excavations, scientists believe that the first winemakers used jars with clay stoppers that helped control the fermentation process.

A complete analysis of the residue left in those ancient wine jugs also showed the presence of terebinth tree resin, which acts as a natural preservative and therefore would have helped slow the transformation of wine into vinegar. In Neolithic times, terebinth trees grew in the same area as grapes, and their berries and resin were harvested at the same time of year. It's quite plausible that some of the berries or resins may have inadvertently become mixed with the grape harvest. Still unclear is whether the ancient winemakers ever made the connection between the resins and the delayed conversion of wine into vinegar and began purposely adding the tree berries to their wine.

Varieties of Vinegar

You might be surprised to learn that there are dozens of types of vinegar. The most common vinegars found in American kitchens are white distilled and apple cider, but the more adventurous may also use red wine vinegar, white wine vinegar, rice vinegar, or gourmet varieties, such as 25-year-old balsamic vinegar or rich black fig vinegar.

As you've learned, vinegar can be made from just about any food that contains natural sugars. Yeast ferments these sugars into alcohol, and certain types of bacteria convert that alcohol a second time into vinegar. A weak acetic acid remains after this second fermentation; the acid has flavors reminiscent of the original fermented food, such as apples or grapes. Acetic acid is what gives vinegar its distinct tart taste. Pure acetic acid can be made in a laboratory; when diluted with water, it is sometimes sold as white vinegar.

However, acetic acids created in labs lack the subtle flavors found in true vinegars, and synthesized versions don't hold a candle to vinegars fermented naturally from summer's sugar-laden fruits or from other foods. Vinegars can be made from many different foods that add their own tastes to the final products, but additional ingredients, such as herbs, spices, or fruits, can be added for further flavor enhancement.

Vinegar is great for a healthy, light style of cooking. The tangy taste often reduces the need for salt, especially in soups and bean dishes. It can also cut the fat in a recipe because it balances flavors without requiring the addition of as much cream, butter, or oil. Vinegar flavors range from mild to bold, so you're sure to find one with the taste you want. A brief look at some of the various vinegars available may help you choose a new one for your culinary escapades.

White Vinegar

This clear variety is the most common type of vinegar in American households. It is made either from grain-based ethanol or laboratory-produced acetic acid and then diluted with water. Its flavor is a bit too harsh for most cooking uses, but it is good for pickling and performing many cleaning jobs around the house.

Wine Vinegar

This flavorful type of vinegar is made from a blend of either red wines or white wines and is common in Europe, especially Germany. Creative cooks often infuse wine vinegars with extra flavor by tucking in a few sprigs. of well-washed fresh herbs, dried herbs, or fresh berries. Red wine vinegar is often flavored with natural raspberry flavoring, if not with the fruit itself.

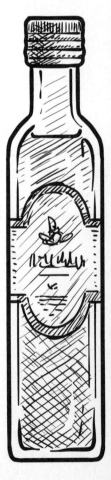

The quality of the original wine determines how good the vinegar is. Better wine vinegars are made from good wines and are aged for a couple of years or more in wooden casks. The result is a fuller, more complex, and mellow flavor. You might find sherry vinegar on the shelf next to the wine vinegars. This variety is made from sherry wine and is usually imported from Spain. Champagne vinegar (yes, made from the bubbly stuff) is a specialty vinegar and is quite expensive.

Apple Cider Vinegar

Apple cider vinegar is the second-most-common type of vinegar in the United States. This light-tan vinegar made from apple cider adds a tart and subtle fruity flavor to your cooking. Along with its health uses, apple cider vinegar is best for salads, dressings, marinades, condiments, and most general vinegar needs.

Traditional Balsamic Vinegar

Traditional balsamic vinegars are artisanal foods, similar to great wines, with long histories and well-developed customs for their production. An excellent balsamic vinegar can be made only by an experienced crafter who has spent many years tending the vinegar, patiently watching and learning.

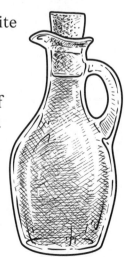

The luscious white and sugary trebbiano grapes that are grown in the northern region of Italy near Modena form the base of the world's best and only true balsamic vinegars. Custom dictates that the grapes be left on the vine for as long as possible to develop their sugar. The juice (or "must") is pressed out of the grapes and boiled down; then, vinegar production begins.

Traditional balsamic vinegar is aged for a number of years—typically 6 and as many as 25. Aging takes place in a succession of casks made from a variety of woods, such as chestnut, mulberry, oak, juniper, and cherry. Each producer has its own formula for the order in which the vinegar is moved to the different casks. Thus, the flavors are complex, rich, sweet, and subtly woody. Vinegar made in this way carries a seal from the Consortium of Producers of the Traditional Balsamic Vinegar of Modena.

Rice Vinegar

Clear or very pale yellow, rice vinegar originated in Japan, where it is essential to sushi preparation. Rice vinegar is made from the sugars found in rice, and the aged, filtered final product has a mild, clean, and delicate flavor that is an excellent complement to ginger or cloves, sometimes with the addition of sugar.

Rice vinegar also comes in red and black varieties, which are not common in the United States but very popular in China. Both are stronger than the clear (often called white) or pale yellow types. Red rice vinegar's flavor is a combination of sweet and tart. Black rice vinegar is common in southern Chinese cooking and has a strong, almost smoky flavor. Rice vinegar is popular in Asian cooking and is great sprinkled on salads and stir-fry dishes. Its gentle flavor is perfect for fruits and tender vegetables, too. Many cooks choose white rice vinegar for their recipes because it does not change the color of the food to which it is added.

Malt Vinegar

This dark-brown vinegar, a favorite in Britain, is reminiscent of deep-brown ale. Malt vinegar production begins with the germination, or sprouting, of barley kernels. Germination enables enzymes to break down starch into sugar. The resulting product is brewed into an alcohol-containing malt beverage or ale. After bacteria convert the ale to vinegar, the vinegar is aged. As its name implies, malt vinegar has a distinctive malt flavor. A cheaper and less flavorful version of malt vinegar consists merely of acetic acid diluted to between 4 percent and 8 percent acidity, with a little caramel coloring added.

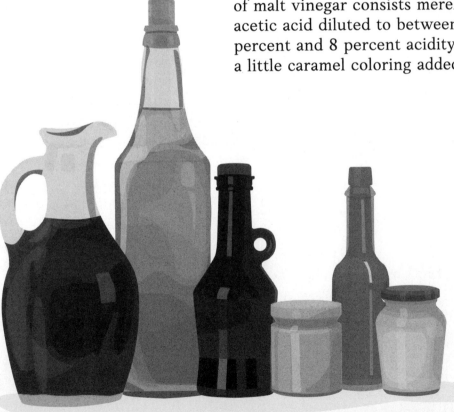

The Benefits of Vinegar in Your Diet

Apple cider vinegar is heralded as a potential healer of many of today's most common serious ailments. Devotees believe vinegar can help prevent or heal heart disease, diabetes, obesity, cancer, aging-related ailments, and a host of other conditions. They say it is full of vitamins, minerals, fiber, enzymes, and pectin and often attribute vinegar's medicinal effects to the presence of these ingredients.

The following are some of the specific claims made about apple cider vinegar:

It reduces blood cholesterol levels and heart-disease risk. Apple cider vinegar fans say it contains pectin, which attaches to cholesterol and carries it out of the body, thus decreasing the risk of heart disease. In addition, many vinegar proponents say it is high in potassium, and high-potassium foods play a role in reducing the risk of heart disease by helping to prevent or lower high blood pressure. Calcium is also an important nutrient for keeping blood pressure in check, and vinegar is sometimes promoted as having a high calcium content. Many also claim vinegar helps the body absorb this essential mineral from other foods in the diet.

It treats diabetes. Apple cider vinegar may help control blood sugar levels, which helps to ward off diabetes complications, such as nerve damage and blindness. It also might help prevent other serious health problems, such as heart disease, that often go hand-in-hand with diabetes.

It fights obesity and aids in weight loss. Some marketers proclaim that apple cider vinegar is high in fiber and therefore aids in weight loss. (Fiber provides bulk but is indigestible by the body, so foods high in fiber provide a feeling of fullness for fewer calories.) A daily dose is also said to control or minimize the appetite. (Ironically, some folk traditions advise taking apple cider vinegar before a meal for the opposite effect—to stimulate the appetite in people who have lost interest in eating.)

It prevents cancer and aging. Apple cider vinegar proponents declare it contains high levels of the antioxidant beta-carotene (a form of vitamin A) and therefore helps prevent cancer and the ill effects of aging. (Antioxidants help protect the body's cells against damage from unstable molecules called free radicals; free-radical damage has been linked to various conditions, including coronary heart disease, cancer, and the aging process.)

It prevents osteoporosis. Advocates say apple cider vinegar releases calcium and other minerals from the foods you eat so your body is better able to absorb and use them to strengthen bones. Vinegar allegedly allows the body to absorb one-third more calcium from green vegetables than it would without the aid of vinegar. Some fans also say apple cider vinegar is itself a great source of calcium. Based on these claims, apple cider vinegar certainly seems to be a wonder food. And it's understandably tempting to want to believe that some food or drug or substance will make diabetes, obesity, cancer, and osteoporosis go away with little or no discomfort, effort, or risk.

However, as a wise consumer, you know that when something sounds too good to be true, it almost certainly is. When it comes to your health—especially when you're dealing with such major medical conditions—it's im-

portant to take a step back and look carefully at the evidence.

A Closer Look at the Claims

With such dramatic claims made for it, you would think that vinegar would be high on the lists of medical researchers searching for the next breakthrough. Yet in the past 20 years, there has been very little research into the use of vinegar for therapeutic health purposes. Granted, a lack of supporting scientific research is a common problem with many natural and alternative therapies. But even the National Center for Complementary and Alternative Medicine (NCCAM), a division of the U.S. government's National Institutes of Health that was created specifically to investigate natural or unconventional therapies that hold promise, has not published any studies about vinegar, despite the fact that there has been renewed interest in vinegar's healing benefits recently.

So, without solid scientific studies, can we judge whether vinegar provides the kinds of dramatic benefits that its promoters and fans attribute to it? Not conclusively. But we can look at the claims and compare them to the little scientific knowledge we do have about vinegar. Those who have faith in apple cider vinegar as a wide-ranging cure say its healing properties come from an abundance of nutrients that remain after apples are fermented to make apple cider vinegar. They contend that vinegar is rich in minerals and vitamins, including calcium, potassium, and beta-carotene; complex carbohydrates and fiber, including the soluble fiber pectin; amino acids (the building blocks of protein); beneficial enzymes; and acetic acid (which gives vinegar its taste).

These substances do play many important roles in health and healing, and some are even considered essential nutrients for human health. The problem is that standard nutritional analysis of vinegar, including apple cider vinegar, has not shown it to be a good source of most of these substances.

Do apple cider vinegar's secrets lie in the vitamins it contains? No. According to the USDA, apple cider vinegar contains no vitamin A, vitamin B6, vitamin C, vitamin E, vitamin K, thiamin, riboflavin, niacin, pantothenic acid, or folate.

What about some of the other health boosting substances that are alleged to be in vinegar? According to detailed nutritional analyses, apple cider vinegar contains no significant amounts of amino acids. Nor does it contain ethyl alcohol, caffeine, theobromine, betacarotene, alpha-carotene, beta-cryptoxanthin, lycopene, lutein, or zeaxanthin.

How Vinegar Can Help

If vinegar doesn't actually contain all the substances that are supposed to account for its medicinal benefits, does that mean it has no healing powers? Hardly. As mentioned, so little research has been done on vinegar that we can't totally rule out many of the dramatic claims made it.

Although we know vinegar doesn't contain loads of nutrients traditionally associated with good health, it may well contain yet-to-be-identified phytochemicals (beneficial compounds in plants) that would account for some of the healing benefits that vinegar fans swear by. Scientists continue to discover such beneficial substances in all kinds of foods.

But beyond that possibility, there appear to be more tangible and realistic—albeit less sensational—ways that vinegar can help the body heal. Rather than being the dramatic blockbuster cure that we are endlessly (and fruitlessly) searching for, vinegar seems quite capable of playing myriad supporting roles—as part of an overall lifestyle approach—that can help us fight serious health conditions, such as osteoporosis, diabetes, and heart disease.

Increasing Calcium Absorption

If there is one thing vinegar fans, marketers, alternative therapists, and scientists alike can agree on, it's that vinegar is high in acetic acid. And acetic acid, like other acids, can increase the body's absorption of important minerals from the foods we eat. Therefore, including apple cider vinegar in meals or possibly even drinking a mild tonic of vine-

gar and water (up to a tablespoon of vinegar in a glass of water) just before or with meals might improve your body's ability to absorb the essential minerals locked in foods.

Vinegar may be especially useful to women, who generally have a hard time getting all the calcium their bodies need to keep bones strong and prevent the debilitating, bone-thinning disease osteoporosis. Although dietary calcium is most abundant in dairy products such as milk, many women (and men) suffer from a condition called lactose intolerance that makes it difficult or impossible for them to digest the sugar in milk. As a result, they may suffer uncomfortable gastrointestinal symptoms, such as cramping and diarrhea, when they consume dairy products.

These women must often look elsewhere to fulfill their dietary calcium needs. Dark, leafy greens are good sources of calcium, but some of these greens also contain compounds that inhibit calcium absorption. Fortunately for dairy-deprived women (and even those who do drink milk), a few splashes of vinegar or a tangy vinaigrette on their greens may very well allow them to absorb more valuable calcium.

Controlling Blood Sugar Levels

Vinegar has recently won attention for its potential to help people with type 2 diabetes get a better handle on their disease. Improved control could help them delay or prevent such complications as blindness, impotence, and a loss of feeling in the extremities that may necessitate amputation.

Also, because people with diabetes are at increased risk for other serious health problems, such as heart disease, improved control of their diabetes could potentially help to ward off these associated conditions, as well.

With type 2 diabetes, the body's cells become resistant to the action of the hormone insulin. The body normally releases insulin into the bloodstream in response to a meal. Insulin's job is to help the body's cells take in the glucose, or sugar, from the carbohydrates in food, so they can use it for energy. But when the body's cells become insulin resistant, sugar from food begins to build up in the blood, even while the cells themselves are starving for it. (High levels of insulin tend to build up in the blood, too, because the body releases more and more insulin to try to transport the large amounts of sugar out of the bloodstream and into the cells.)

Over time, high levels of blood sugar can damage nerves throughout the body and otherwise cause irreversible harm. One major goal of diabetes treatment is to normalize blood sugar levels and keep them in a healthier range as much as possible. And that's where vinegar appears to help.

It seems that vinegar may be able to inactivate some of the digestive enzymes that break the carbohydrates from food into sugar, thus slowing the absorption of sugar from a meal into the bloodstream. Slowing sugar absorption gives the insulin-resistant body more time to pull sugar out of the blood and thus helps prevent the blood sugar level from rising so high. Blunting the sudden jump in blood sugar that would usually occur after a meal also lessens the amount of insulin the body needs to release at one time to remove the sugar from the blood.

A study cited in 2004 in the American Diabetes Association's publication *Diabetes Care* indicates that vinegar holds real promise for helping people with diabetes. In the study, 21 people with either type 2 diabetes or insulin resistance (a prediabetic condition) and 8 control subjects were each given a solution containing five teaspoons of vinegar, five teaspoons of water, and one teaspoon of saccharin two minutes before ingesting a high-carbohydrate meal.

The blood sugar and insulin levels of the participants were measured before the meal and 30 minutes and 60 minutes after the meal. Vinegar increased overall insulin sensitivity 34 percent in the study participants

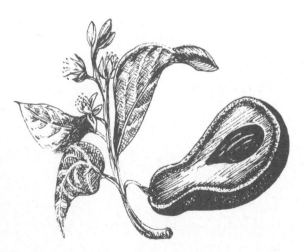

who were insulin-resistant and 19 percent in those with type 2 diabetes. That means their bodies actually became more receptive to insulin, allowing the hormone to do its job of getting sugar out of the blood and into the cells. Both blood sugar and blood insulin levels were lower than usual in the insulin-resistant participants, which is more good news.

Surprisingly, the control group (who had neither diabetes nor a prediabetic condition but were given the vinegar solution) also experienced a reduction in insulin levels in the blood. These findings are significant because, in addition to the nerve damage caused by perpetually elevated blood sugar levels, several chronic conditions, including heart disease, have been linked to excess insulin in the blood over prolonged periods of time.

More studies certainly need to be done to confirm the extent of vinegar's benefits for type 2 diabetes patients and those at risk of developing this increasingly common disease. But for now, people with type 2 diabetes might be wise to talk with their doctors or dietitians about consuming more vinegar.

Replacing Unhealthy Fats and Sodium

There are some delicious varieties of vinegar available—and you're not limited to apple cider vinegar to get the benefits! Each bestows a different taste or character on foods. The diversity and intensity of flavor are key to one important healing role that vinegar can play. Whether you are trying to protect yourself from cardiovascular diseases, such as heart disease, high blood pressure, or stroke, or you have been diagnosed with one or more of these conditions and have been advised to clean up your diet, vinegar should become a regular cooking and dining companion.

That's because a tasty vinegar can often be used in place of sodium and/or ingredients high in saturated or trans fats to add flavor and excitement to a variety of dishes. Saturated and trans fats have been shown to have a detrimental effect on blood cholesterol levels, and experts recommend that people who have or are at risk of developing high blood pressure cut back on the amount of sodium they consume. Using vinegar as a simple, flavorful substitute

for these less healthful ingredients as often as possible can help people manage blood cholesterol and blood pressure levels and, in turn, help ward off heart disease and stroke.

Removing Harmful Substances from Produce

Some people are concerned that eating large amounts of fruits and vegetables may lead to an unhealthy consumption of pesticides and other farm-chemical residues. Vinegar can lend a hand here, too. Washing produce in a mixture of water and vinegar appears to help remove certain pesticides, according to the small amount of research that has been published. Vinegar also appears to be helpful in getting rid of harmful bacteria on fruits and vegetables.

To help remove potentially harmful residues, mix a solution of 10 percent vinegar to 90 percent water (for example, mix one cup of white vinegar in nine cups of water). Then, place produce in the vinegar solution, let it soak briefly, and then swish it around in the solution. Finally, rinse the produce thoroughly. Do not use this process on tender, fragile fruits, such as berries, that might be damaged in the process or soak up too much vinegar through their porous skins. Some pesticide residues are trapped beneath the waxy coatings that are applied to certain vegetables to help them retain moisture. The vinegar solution probably won't wash those pesticides away, so peeling lightly may be a better option. Some research suggests that cooking further eliminates some pesticide residue.

Should You Supplement?

Some people believe in the healing power of apple cider vinegar but would rather take it in tablet form instead of using it as a daily tonic or adding it to food. But like any shortcut on the road to better health, you can't be sure this one will get you to the goal you're aiming for.

Part of the reason for concern is that the U.S. Food and Drug Administration (FDA) does not regulate supplements, so you really can't be  sure what you're getting. In a study reported in the July 2005 *Journal of* *the American Dietetic Association,* for example, researchers analyzed eight different brands of apple cider vinegar tablets. The analysis showed most had acetic acid levels different from those claimed on the label. How much of a problem is this? Well, it would be natural to think the more acetic acid the better. But in truth, at a level of 11 percent, acetic acid can cause burns to the skin. And at 20 percent, it is considered poisonous. Some of the analyzed supplements, however, claimed to contain a frightening 35 percent acetic acid!

Fortunately for their users, none did. The acetic acid content actually ranged from 1.04 percent to 10.57 percent. Another reason to go natural: Several of the samples were contaminated with mold and/or yeast, including one that claimed to be yeast-free. In addition, because so little scientific research has been done to verify the healing claims made for vinegar— and the possible ingredients or actions that might be responsible—it's impossible to know if supplements would have the same effects as the real thing. Indeed, most of vinegar's benefits—at least the ones that rest on the most solid scientific grounds—are those based on its use as a substitute for unhealthy ingredients in the diet, a role that simply could not be played by a pill.

At this time, it would seem you are almost certainly better off including more vinegar in your diet, taking advantage of its potential healing benefits as well as its phenomenal flavors, rather than spending more money on supplements that may not have any benefit and could even be dangerous.

Apple Cider Vinegar Remedies

The use of vinegar as medicine probably started soon after it was discovered. Its healing virtues are extolled in records of the Babylonians, and the great Greek physician Hippocrates reportedly used it as an antibiotic. Ancient Greek doctors poured vinegar into wounds and over dressings as a disinfectant, and they gave concoctions of honey and vinegar to patients recovering from illness. In Asia, early samurai warriors believed vinegar to be a tonic that would increase their strength and vitality.

Vinegar has continued to be used as a medicine in more recent times. During the Civil War and World War I, for example, military medics used vinegar to treat wounds. Folk traditions around the world still espouse vinegar for a wide variety of ailments. Natural healing enthusiasts and vinegar fans continue to honor and use many of those folk remedies. Vinegar's potential for treating or preventing major medical problems is of interest to almost everyone.

But apple cider vinegar in particular has also has been cherished as a home remedy for some common minor ailments for centuries. In this chapter, we'll look at some of those conditions and suggested remedies. Although they're not life-or-death issues, these minor health problems can be uncomfortable, and there is often little modern medicine can offer in the way of a cure. So you may want to give apple cider vinegar a shot to determine for yourself if it can help. (It's always best when trying any remedy for the first time to run it past your doctor to be sure there is no reason you should not try it.)

Muscle Aches

The vast array of muscles in your body is what allows you to do something as simple as picking up a fork or as complicated as a kickboxing routine. Muscles are a complex weave of fibers that work with your brain and skeletal system to give you the agility to return that volley across the tennis court. When you're taking care to stretch and strengthen your muscles, they are your greatest ally. But when they don't work like they should or they get injured, you end up with a very painful problem on your hands.

Strains are one of the most common reasons for aching muscles. When you strain a muscle, it means you've worked it too hard, causing the muscle fibers to pull and tear. If you haven't worked out for a while and then head back full throttle without preparing your muscles for the trauma they're about to experience, or if you're an experienced exerciser and you don't warm up properly, you risk getting a strained muscle. At best, a strained muscle will leave you sore for a few days; at worst, you could end up with a "pulled" muscle, one whose fibers have been totally torn. Another common muscle malady is cramps, or

spasms. Muscle cramps happen when the muscle isn't getting enough blood, and in response to the restricted blood flow the muscle shortens and tightens. The slowdown in blood flow can be caused by a variety of problems.

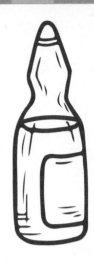

Remedies:

Add 1 cup apple cider vinegar to a bathtub of warm water. Soak in tub for at least 15 minutes.

Boil 1 cup apple cider vinegar and add 1 teaspoon ground red pepper during boil. Cool this mixture, then apply it in a compress to sore area. Make sure pepper doesn't irritate the skin. The compress should make the area feel warm but not burning.

Try this liniment during a rubdown to relieve achy muscles and arthritis pain: Mix 1 cup apple cider vinegar, 1 cup extra virgin olive oil, and 2 egg whites. Massage into the painful parts; use a clean cotton cloth to wipe off any excess.

In folk medicine some herbs have been labeled "counterirritants." These herbs stimulate blood flow to the skin and the muscles underneath. One common counterirritant in folk healing is mustard seeds. Try this mustard plaster when your muscles ache.

❧ Crush the seeds of white or brown mustard.

❧ Moisten with vinegar and sprinkle with flour.

❧ Spread mixture on a cloth, and cover with a second cloth.

❧ Lay the moist side on the painful area, and leave on for 20 minutes. (Remove the plaster if it becomes painful.)

Athlete's Foot

Athlete's foot itches, burns, and is downright ugly to look at. But it's not a condition unique to athletes. Blame the misnomer on the ad man who gave it its name in the 1930s. In fact, athlete's foot, or *tinea pedis*, is the most common fungal infection of the skin. This fungus loves moist places, especially the soft, warm, damp skin between the toes. Certainly, the athlete's locker room environment, with its steamy showers, is a good place for the fungus to thrive. But *tinea pedis* is actually present on most people's skin all the time, just waiting for the right opportunity to develop into an infection.

So what causes athlete's foot to rear its ugly little fungal head? Skin that's irritated, weakened, or continuously moist is primed for an athlete's foot infection. And certain medications, including antibiotics, corticosteroids, birth control pills, and drugs that suppress immune function, can make you more susceptible. People who are obese and those who have diabetes mellitus or a weakened immune system, such as those with AIDS, also are at increased risk. And some people may be genetically pre-disposed to developing athlete's foot.

Anyone can get athlete's foot—and most people will at some time in their lives. Teenage and adult males, though, are the most susceptible. People who spend a lot of time barefoot, women, and children under the age of 12 have the lowest risk.

Remedies:
Mix equal parts apple cider (or regular) vinegar and ethyl alcohol. Dab on the affected areas.

Create an environment that is inhospitable to the fungus that causes the condition. The Amish traditionally use a footbath of vinegar and water to discourage the growth of athlete's foot fungus. To try this remedy, mix one cup of vinegar into two quarts of water in a basin or pan. Soak your feet in this solution every night for 15 to 30 minutes, using a fresh solution each night.

Or, if you prefer, mix up a solution using one cup of vinegar and one cup of water. Apply the solution to the affected parts of your feet with a cotton ball. Let your feet dry completely before putting on socks and/or shoes.

Bug Bites

With billions of bugs out there, you're bound to get bit or stung sometime in your life. Typically, the worst reactions are to bees, yellow jackets, hornets, wasps, and fire ants. Other nasty creatures, such as blackflies, horseflies, black or red (not fire) ants, and mosquitoes, also bite and sting, but their venom usually does not cause as intense a reaction. No matter who attacks, once you're zapped the body reacts with redness, itching, pain, and swelling at the bite site. These symptoms may last for a few minutes or a few hours. Thankfully, relief is as close as the kitchen. **Warning!** These remedies only apply to bites and stings from insects. A health provider should treat those

from snakes, spiders, scorpions, ticks, centipedes, and animals. If the person bitten has a known allergy to insect venom or begins to exhibit signs of a serious allergic reaction, such as widespread hives, swelling of the face or mouth, difficulty breathing, or loss of consciousness, skip the home remedies and seek immediate medical attention.

Remedies:
No matter whether it's the white or the apple cider variety, vinegar turns insect sting pain into a thing of the past. Mix one tablespoon each of vinegar and baking soda. Apply the paste, and leave it on the sting as long as possible. Apply more, if necessary.

You can also use vinegar mixed with cornstarch to make a paste. Apply paste to a bee sting or bug bite and let dry.

Bronchitis

That nasty cold has been hanging on much longer than it should, and day by day it seems to be getting worse. Your chest hurts, you gurgle when you breathe, and you're coughing so much yellow, green, or gray mucus that your throat is raw. These symptoms are letting you know that your cold has probably turned into a respiratory infection called bronchitis, an inflammation of the little branches and tubes of your windpipe that also makes them swell. No wonder breathing has become such a chore. Your air passages are too puffy to carry air very easily.

Acute bronchitis can include these other symptoms, too:

- Wheezing
- Shortness of breath
- Fever or chills
- General aches and pains
- Upper chest pain

Bronchitis is not contagious since it's a secondary infection that develops when your immune system is weakened by a cold or the flu. Some people are prone to developing it, some are not. Those at the top of the risk list have respiratory problems already, such as asthma, allergies, and emphysema. People who have a weakened immune system also are more prone to bronchitis. But anyone can develop it, and most people do at one time or another.

Remedies:

The xanthine derivatives in coffee are good bronchodilators. To cut down on mucus problems, add 1 teaspoon apple cider vinegar and 2 drops peppermint oil to a cup of black coffee, either instant or brewed. Drink 1 cup in the morning and evening.

Colds

Every year Americans will suffer through more than one billion colds. That's one billion runny noses, coughs, sneezes, aches, and sore throats. Colds make such frequent appearances that the infection has come to be known as the "common cold." Small children are the most likely to catch a cold: Most kids will have six to ten colds a year. That's because their young immune systems combined with the germy confines of school and daycare situations make them prime targets for the virus. The upside of having so many colds as a child is that you develop immunities to some of the 200 viruses that cause colds. As a result, adults get an average of only two to four colds a year. By the time most people reach age 60, they're down to about one cold per year. Women, however, especially women between 20 and 30 years old, get more colds than men.

Remedies:

For a sore throat, mix one teaspoon of apple cider vinegar into a glass of water; gargle with a mouthful of the solution and then swallow it, repeating until you've finished all the solution in the glass.

For a natural cough syrup, mix half a tablespoon apple cider vinegar with half a tablespoon honey and swallow. Or mix 1/4 cup honey and apple cider vinegar; pour into a jar or bottle that can be tightly sealed. Shake well before each use. Take 1 tablespoon every 4 hours. If cough persists for more than a week, see a physician. (Do not give it or any other honey-containing food or beverage to children younger than two years of age. Honey can carry a bacterium that can cause a kind of food poisoning called infant botulism and may also cause allergic reactions in very young children.)

You can add a quarter-cup of apple cider vinegar to the recommended amount of water in your room vaporizer to help with congestion. To alleviate a sore throat and also thin mucus, gargle with apple cider vinegar that has a little salt and ground black pepper added to it.

Fever

Fever is a good thing. It's your body's attempt to kill off invading bacteria and other nasty organisms that can't survive the heat. The hypothalamus, which is the body's thermostat, senses the assault on the body and turns up the heat much the way you turn up the thermostat when you feel cold. It's a simple defense mechanism, and the sweat that comes with a fever is merely a way to cool the body down.

It used to be standard medical practice to knock that fever out as quickly as possible. Not so anymore. The value of fever is recognized, and since a fever will usually subside when the infection that's causing it runs its course, modern thinking is to ride out that fever, especially if it stays under 102 degrees Fahrenheit in adults. However, if a fever is making you uncomfortable or interfering with your ability to eat, drink, or sleep, treat it. Your body needs adequate nutrition, hydration, and rest to fight the underlying cause of the fever.

Fever is a symptom, not an illness, and so there's no specific cure. But there is one traditional remedy involving vinegar that may help you feel better.

Remedies:

Blackberry vinegar is a great fever elixir, but it takes several days to prepare. Pour cider vinegar over a pound or two of blackberries, then cover the container and store it in a cool, dark place for three days. Strain for a day, since it takes time for all the liquid to drain from the berries, and collect the liquid in another container. Then add 2 cups sugar to each 2.5 cups juice. Bring to a boil, then simmer for 5 minutes while you skim the scum off the top. Cool and store in an airtight jar in a cool place. Mix 1 teaspoonful with water to quench the thirst caused by a fever.

Headaches

The day starts with screaming kids, continues slowly onward with stop 'n' go traffic, and ends on a sour note with an angry boss. By this point, you are ready to chop your head off in order to relieve the pounding pain. You can take a little comfort in knowing that almost everyone has had such a day...and such a headache. Yet some people fare worse than others do. An estimated 45 million Americans get chronic, recurring headaches, while as many as 18 million of those suffer from painful, debilitating migraines.

Remedies:

Ease a headache by lying down and applying a compress dipped in a mixture of half warm water and half apple cider vinegar to the temples. Use above treatment for treating a headache, but try an herbal vinegar such as lavender to provide aromatic relief.

If you suffer from recurring headaches, you might want to plant a little feverfew in your herb garden (or grow the herb in a windowsill pot). This lovely, easy-to-nurture herb has long been used as a headache remedy, especially for migraines. Feverfew causes blood vessels to dilate and inhibits the secretion of substances that cause pain and inflammation (such as histamine and serotonin) through the substance parthenolide. You have two choices when it comes to taking feverfew: eating it raw or drinking it in tea. If you do prefer the au naturel way, add 2 to 3 of the leaves to a salad dressed with vinegar.

Heartburn

Boy, oh boy, did you do it this time. You added that heaping second helping to all the platter pickings you couldn't resist, and what do you have? Indigestion (an incomplete or imperfect digestion), that's what. And it may be accompanied by pain, nausea, vomiting, heartburn, gas, and belching. All this because you couldn't resist temptation. But don't worry. It happens to everybody, and it goes away.

So, now that you've eaten until you're about ready to burst, what's next? The couch, maybe? Stretch out, let your digestive system do its thing, take a nap? Wrong! The worst thing you can do after a binge is to lie down. That can cause heartburn, also known as acid indigestion. Whatever you call it, it's

the feeling you get when digestive acid escapes your stomach and irritates the esophagus, the tube that leads from your throat to your stomach. After you eat, heartburn can also fire up when you exercise, bend forward, or strain muscles.

Remedies:

There are several prescription medicines available for the treatment of long-term or serious heartburn or acid reflux, and over-the-counter remedies are available at your pharmacy, too. But you can also try this home remedy. Mix 1 tablespoon apple cider vinegar, 1 tablespoon honey, and 1 cup warm water. Drink at the first sign of heartburn.

Itches

To scratch or not to scratch, that is the question. When confronted with an itch, most of us tend to throw self-discipline out the door and scratch to our skin's content. While that may prove momentarily satisfying, scratching excessively can injure your skin. And if you break the skin, you leave yourself open to infection. Itching, medically known as pruritus, is caused by stimuli bugging some part of our skin. There are a lot of places to bother on the body, too. The average adult has 20 square feet (2 square meters) of skin, all open to the world of irritants. When something bothers our skin, an itch is a built-in defense mechanism that alerts the body that someone is knocking. We respond to an itch with a scratch, as most people want to remove the problem. But the scratching can also set you up for the "itch-scratch" cycle, where one leads to the other endlessly.

An itch can range from a mild nuisance to a disrupting, damaging, and sleep-depriving fiasco. Itches happen for many reasons, including allergic reactions; sunburns; insect bites; poison ivy; reactions to chemicals, soaps, and detergents; medication; dry weather; skin infections; and even aging. More serious itches, such as those caused by psoriasis or other diseases, are not covered here. Fortunately, scratching isn't the only solution to an itch.

Remedies:

To relieve itchy skin, add 1 cup apple cider vinegar to a bathtub of warm water. Soak in tub for at least 15 minutes.

Use your freezer to soothe and cool just about any kind of skin itchiness, be it from sunburn, a bug bite, or a rash. Fill each compartment of an empty, clean foam egg carton with apple cider vinegar; freeze. When the itch gets insane, pop out a vinegar cube and rub it over the spot.

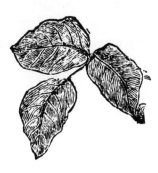

Laryngitis

Have you been verbally abusing your voice? Too much vocal enthusiasm at a sports event can set you up for swollen vocal cords and no voice the next day. But that's not the only way to cause laryngitis—the result of inflammation of the voice box and voice folds. More often, laryngitis is caused by an upper respiratory infection, usually viral, such as the common cold. Surprisingly, some cases of laryngitis are caused by heartburn, especially in the elderly. During the night, the acid-rich contents of the stomach come back up the throat and cause irritation.

Remedies:

Viruses and bacteria dread an acidic environment, so why not make your mouth one big, albeit weak, acid bath? Gargling with vinegar, a weak acid, can help wipe out many infectious organisms. Pour equal amounts of vinegar and water into a cup, mix, and gargle two to four times a day. You can also gargle with straight vinegar, but some people find it too strong, especially at first.

Laryngitis can be caused by a viral infection and is easily spread by hand-to-hand contact or by touching contaminated surfaces. Avoiding such germs is one of the best ways to prevent laryngitis. If you or someone around you has a cold, be extra vigilant about washing your hands with warm water and soap. Clean common surfaces, such as the telephone and door handles, with vinegar and a clean cloth.

Poison Ivy

Contact with poison ivy, poison oak, or poison sumac often goes hand-in-hand with camping and other outdoor activities. Outdoor enthusiasts by the tentful have had to cut trips short after an unfortunate encounter with any one of this painful threesome. The problem stems from the plant's colorless oil called urushiol. Whenever one of these plants is cut, crushed, stepped on, sat on, grabbed, rolled on, kicked, or disturbed, the oil is released. Once on the victim, the toxic oil penetrates the skin and a rash appears within 12 to 48 hours after exposure. This is a true allergic reaction to compounds in the urushiol. The rash starts as small bumps and progresses into enlarged, itchy blisters. No body part is immune to the oil, although areas most often irritated are the face, arms, hands, legs, and genitals.

Remedies:
Be it from plant, insect, or allergic reaction, itches of all sorts are tamed by a simple vinegar rinse. First wash the affected area with soap and lukewarm water, then rinse. Apply vinegar with a cotton ball, rub gently, and rinse.

Before going to bed, pour a cup of baking soda into a lukewarm bath and take a soak.

Psoriasis

Psoriasis is a noncontagious, chronic skin condition that produces round, dry, scaly patches that are covered with white, gray, or silver-white scales. These patches are called plaques. Although psoriasis is a mysterious condition (doctors aren't exactly sure what causes it or why it can be mild one day and serious the next), it is common. According to information from the National Institutes of Health, between 5.8 million and 7.5 million Americans have the disease. Psoriasis is also tough to treat because what works for one person may not work for another, and treatments that were once effective for an individual often become ineffective, and vice versa.

Remedies:

One solution that some people have found helpful to try is an apple cider vinegar dip. It's a great soak for affected fingernails and toenails; just pour some in a bowl or cup and dip your nails in for a few minutes. Some people have also had success applying it to plaques using cotton balls.

Sunburn

A sunburn is one of the most common hazards of the great outdoors. The unappealing and painful lobster look results when the amount of exposure to the sun exceeds the ability of the body's protective pigment, melanin, to protect the skin. What makes sunburn different from, say, a household iron burn? A sunburn is not immediately apparent. By the time the skin starts to become red, the damage has been done. Pain isn't always instantly noticeable, either.

You may feel glowing after two hours sitting poolside without sun protection. But just wait awhile. You'll change your tune (not to mention color) when the pain sets in, typically 6 to 48 hours after sun exposure. Like household burns, sunburns are summed up by degree. Mild sunburns are deep pink, punctuated by a hot, burning sensation. Moderate sunburns are red, clothing lines are prominent, and the skin itches and stings. Severe sunburns result in bright red skin, blisters, fever, chills, and nausea.

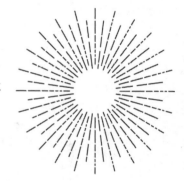

Remedies:

A mixture of white or apple cider vinegar with an equal amount of cool water can be used to bathe a garden variety sunburn. If no one is around to help you, fill a spray bottle with the solution and spray the affected areas. You can also wear a large, loose-fitting soft cotton T-shirt that has been soaked in the mixture.

Toothaches

We take those choppers for granted, don't we? Except for that first year or two of life, they've always been there, ready to take on the grueling task of chewing. We douse them with sugar that erodes their enamel, require them to work overtime on foods hard enough to be called petrified, and then we forget the basics our parents taught us: Brush after every meal, and don't eat so many sweets. Our teeth serve us well when they're in good order, but when something goes wrong, ouch!

First comes that off-and-on-again little twinge, the one we ignore and hope will disappear. Next comes the sensitivity to hot and cold. And finally, the full-out throb that hurts so bad that pulling the tooth out with a piece of string tied to a doorknob doesn't seem like such a bad way out.

Tooth problems hurt and ultimately the solution comes in a dentist's chair, the drill screaming in your ear, your teeth clenching against the needle being jabbed into your mouth. Yes, we do abuse our teeth. And what's amazing about that is that overall, we're not neglecting our dental health. On average, 65 percent of all Americans visit their dentist regularly.

So, what's the deal? Why the toothache? Some reasons are:

- Poor food choices
- Bacteria
- Bad brushing technique
- Not enough flossing
- Heredity
- Lack of professional care

But fear not, vinegar can help remedy some of your dental dilemmas, be it a toothache or tooth care in general.

Remedies:
Here's an easy but temporary toothache fix. Try rinsing your mouth with a mixture of 4 ounces warm water, 2 tablespoons apple cider vinegar, and 1 tablespoon salt. If toothache persists, see a dentist.

To brighten dentures, soak them overnight in pure white vinegar.

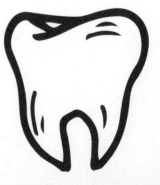

Chapter 3: Soothe Everyday Aches & Pains

Pain

Pain is an unpleasant or uncomfortable sensation that can range from mild irritation to excruciating agony. It is probably the most commonly reported symptom and is linked to innumerable disorders and diseases. Pain occurs when specialized nerve endings are stimulated; within a fraction of a second this pain "signal" travels through a network of nerves to the brain. Pain can be a warning sign, indicating impending damage to the body, or it can be a protective mechanism, causing the person feeling pain to remove the cause or reflexively draw away from the source.

Most healthy people have occasional, brief twinges of pain that have no specific cause and are usually harmless. However, bothersome, recurring, or persistent pain can be caused by thousands of factors. Most commonly, pain is a symptom of disease, injury, or abnormal changes in the body.

There are many types of pain. Pain can be dull and constant, sharp and sudden crushing, burning, piercing, or aching. When it is felt in areas other than the location of the disorder (for example, when the pain of heart attack is felt in the arm), it is called referred pain. Unexplainable pain should be reported promptly to a doctor for investigation to locate its source for it to be treatment.

Using plants to quiet pain goes back before the dawn of recorded medical history, but none of these plants proved particularly effective. That is why this century brought about newer and better pain drugs and why pain medications are among the most popular over-the-counter drugs. Many of the modern drugs, such as aspirin, acetaminophen, ibuprofen, and corticosteroids, suppress the formation of prostaglandins, a class of chemicals in the local tissues that trigger pain. There are other, more potent painkillers, such as the opiates, morphine, and codeine, but these must be prescribed by a doctor.

Many of the plants used in natural medicine for pain relief use the same biochemical pathways as the non-opiate pain-relieving drugs, but they are not as effective. On the other hand, many of these plants have multiple effects. Their antispasmodic and circulation-promoting constituents may make up for what these plants lack in prostaglandin-suppressing strength. Comparative trials of these plants with drugs have not been performed, but the plants' persistent use in natural medicine (even with the availability of inexpensive over-the-counter drugs) indicates that they must have at least some beneficial effect.

Herbal formulas that combine prostaglandin-suppressing, antispasmodic, sedative, and antidepressant plants are commonly prescribed by professional herbalists in North America, Great Britain, and Australia.

Traditions throughout North America and other parts of the world also make use of irritating liniments and plasters to treat muscle and joint pain. These natural remedies are applied externally to irritate the skin over the site of the pain. Physiological tests show that such treatments increase blood flow to the skin by as much as four times and also increase blood flow and temperature in the muscles underneath the skin. Any relief from such treatments is due to this increased circulation to the area, which ensures a healthy flow of oxygen to the tissues and relieves the swelling of stagnant lymph in the area. This method, called counterirritation, may also increase local or systemic levels of endorphins, the body's natural pain-killing substances that are more potent than opiates.

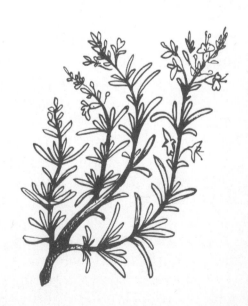

Natural Remedies for Pain

Hot Peppers

Cayenne pepper (*Capsicum* spp.) is used in formulas for liniments and plasters in the natural medicine of China, the American Southwest, Utah, and throughout Ohio, Indiana, and Illinois. External and internal use of cayenne pepper to stimulate circulation was a key element of Thomsonian herbalism throughout rural New England and the Midwest in the early 1800s. (The Thomsonian movement of herbalism was introduced into practice in the early 19th century by Samuel Thomson, an influential New England herbalist. Thomsonian herbalism has been a powerful influence on American herbal traditions for the last 190 years.) Capsaicin, a constituent of cayenne, stimulates pain receptors without actually burning the tissues. Cayenne is thus one of the safest items to use for counterirritation.

You can place one ounce of cayenne pepper in a quart of rubbing alcohol. Let the mixture stand for three weeks, shaking the bottle each day. Then, apply to the affected part during acute attacks.

Alternately, if you can't wait three weeks for relief, try this method: Place one ounce of cayenne pepper in a pint of boiling water. Simmer for half an hour. Do not strain, but add a pint of rubbing alcohol. Let cool to room temperature. Apply as desired to the affected part. (Do not ingest either of these remedies.)

Cramp Bark and Black Haw

For the treatment of spasmodic pain, both cramp bark (*Viburnum opulus*) and black haw (*Viburnum prunifolium*) have been used in American Indian medicine. The Cherokee, Delaware, Fox, and Ojibwa tribes all used cramp bark to treat both menstrual pain and muscle spasm. Cramp bark and black haw were used for arthritic or menstrual pain in Physiomedicalist and Eclectic medicine. The plants contain the antispasmodic and muscle-relaxing compounds esculetin and scopoletin. The antispasmodic constituents are best extracted with alcohol (rather than water), so tinctures may be more effective than teas. Black haw also contains aspirin-like compounds.

Purchase one ounce each of cramp bark and black haw tincture in a health food store or herb shop. If both aren't available, either one will do. Mix them together, and take two droppers every two or three hours for up to three days.

Ginger

Ginger is used to treat various sorts of pain in the medicine of China. It is also used for pain or spasm in the medicine of New England, Appalachia, North Carolina, and Indiana. It is an important pain medication in contemporary Arabic medicine; reports of its use there in treating migraine headache and arthritis show its effectiveness. Ginger contains twelve different aromatic anti-inflammatory compounds, including some with mild aspirin-like effects.

You can cut a fresh ginger root (about the size of your thumb) into thin slices. Place the slices in a quart of water. Bring to a boil, and then simmer on the lowest possible heat for thirty minutes in a covered pot. Let cool for thirty more minutes. Strain and drink one cup, sweetened with honey, as desired.

Epsom Salt Baths

Traditions in both New England and Indiana call for Epsom salt baths to relieve pain. Epsom salt was named after a salt found in abundance in spring water near the town of Epsom, England, in 1618. The salt was reputed to have magical healing properties. Epsom salt is now produced industrially and not from the springs in England. Epsom salt is primarily magnesium sulfate and has been used medicinally in Europe for more than three hundred years. The heat of an Epsom salt bath can increase circulation and reduce the swelling of arthritis, and the magnesium can be absorbed through the skin. Magnesium is one of the most important minerals in the body, participating in at least 300 enzyme systems. Magnesium has both anti-inflammatory and anti-arthritic properties.

Muscle Strains and Sprains

When the body's tissues are injured, the body initiates the process of inflammation to heal them. Blood flow increases to the area, causing redness. Lymph floods the tissues, causing swelling. (The initial flooding of lymph to the area can cause severe pain as the tissues are stretched.) Chemicals that cause pain are secreted to the damaged tissues. The net effect of all this swelling and pain is to immobilize the area to prevent further injury. Next, some of the body's white blood cells migrate to the area to clear away damaged tissue. Good circulation is necessary at this stage to bring in the nutrients necessary to build new tissue and to carry away the debris of the injury. You can decrease the pain in the area by reducing the swelling. Soak the affected part in cool water. After the first day, however, it is important to increase circulation to the injured part. To do this, treat the area with hot soaks and massage.

Folk traditions throughout North America and other parts of the world also make use of counterirritants to treat muscle strains and sprains. Other folk remedies are taken internally and have pharmacological effects similar to aspirin.

Natural Remedies for Strains and Sprains

Mustard Plaster

Mustard plaster, used since the dawn of history, remains today in the medical literature of Appalachia, China, and Europe. The irritating substance in mustard is not activated until the seeds are crushed and mixed with liquid.

Crush the seeds of white mustard (*Brassica alba*) or brown mustard (*Brassica juncea*) or grind them in a seed grinder. Moisten the mixture with vinegar and sprinkle with flour. Spread the mixture on a cloth. Cover with a second cloth. Lay the moist side across the painful area. Leave on about twenty minutes. Remove if the poultice becomes uncomfortable. Wash the affected area.

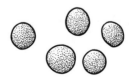

Rosemary

Rosemary (*Rosmarinus officinalis*) was used to relieve pain and spasm by doctors of the Physiomedicalist school in the last century. Today, rosemary is used (both externally and internally) in the natural medicine of Mexico and the Southwest for treating the pain of pulled muscles. Rosemary contains four anti-inflammatory substances, including rosmarinic acid, which has a biochemical action similar to aspirin. Rosmarinic acid is also easily absorbed through the skin and is approved as a topical analgesic by the German government.

Put one ounce of rosemary leaves in a one-pint canning jar and fill with boiling water. Cover tightly and let stand for thirty minutes. Apply as a wash over the painful area two to three times a day.

Wintergreen Oil

Wintergreen (*Gaultheria procumbens*) has been used to treat muscle pain by the Delaware, Menominee, Ojibwa, Potawatomi, and Iroquois Indian tribes. It entered into official United States medicine for this purpose in 1820 and remains, in the form of wintergreen oil, a medicine included in the United States Pharmacopoeia.

Wintergreen and wintergreen oil also appear as treatments for muscle pain in the natural medicine of New England. The active pain-relieving constituent in wintergreen is methyl-salicylate, a chemical relative of aspirin. The concentrated oil has been used as a pain-relieving medicine since the 1800s, but it can be toxic, even when applied to the skin. (Aspirin was discovered during the search for safer pain-relieving drugs.) If you want to use this plant, stick with the dried herb.

You can pour one pint of boiling water over one ounce of dried wintergreen leaves in a cup. Let stand until it reaches room temperature. Apply as a wash over the affected area, and, simultaneously, take two-ounce doses of the tea three to four times a day.

Witch Hazel

Witch hazel is a tree native to North America. It contains both astringent and anti-inflammatory properties. Settlers learned the use of witch hazel for treating pain from the Indians of the Oneida tribe in New York. In the 1840s, the use of the plant spread throughout the United States in the form of various over-the-counter products. The use of witch hazel later spread to

Europe, where its extract became popular. Witch hazel extract remains in use today in professional British herbalism and in conventional German medicine. The German government has approved the use of witch hazel for treating minor inflammations, especially of the skin and mucous membranes. Witch hazel is also used in the natural remedy of New England as an external application for sprains.

Arthritis

In a nutshell, arthritis means "inflammation of the joints." Rheumatism is an old medical term that was used to describe inflammation of either joints or muscles. Rheum was thought to be a watery mucus-like secretion, sometimes brought on by cold weather. Joint or muscle pain was thought to be caused by such secretions trapped in the tissues. Although the concept is not far from the truth–inflammation is usually accompanied by swelling and a build-up of fluid—the modern explanation of arthritis is much more precise.

Today's medical experts suggest there are at least twenty-three varieties of arthritis, including rheumatoid arthritis and osteoarthri-tis, the two most common types. With osteoarthritis—sometimes called degenerative joint disease, or DJD—there is a gradual wearing away of cartilage in the joints. Healthy cartilage is the elastic tissue that lines and cushions the joints and allows bones to move smoothly against one another.

When this cartilage deteriorates, the bones rub together, causing pain and swelling. Permanent damage and stiffness of the joints is possible.

Rheumatoid arthritis can attack at any age. This form of arthritis affects all the connective tissues, as well as other organs. The precise cause of rheumatoid arthritis is unknown. Some researchers believe that a virus triggers the disease, causing an autoimmune response whereby the body attacks its own tissues. However, evidence for this theory is inconclusive. What is confirmed is the progression of the condition. First, the synovium (the thin membrane that lines and lubricates the joint) becomes inflamed.

The inflammation eventually destroys the cartilage. As scar tissue gradually replaces the damaged cartilage, the joint becomes misshaped and rigid. Rheumatoid arthritis may damage the heart, lungs, nerves, eyes, and joints.

A medical examination and diagnosis are required to identify the cause and nature of any chronic joint or muscular pain. Other "rheumatic" diseases include arthralgia (pain in a joint), fibrositis ("muscular rheumatism"), and synovitis (inflammation of the joint membrane).

There is no simple cure for arthritis. Conventional treatment for chronic joint pain is to use drugs to suppress the inflammation in order to reduce pain and also prevent tissue destruction. Usually, simple aspirin-related pain medications, called nonsteroidal anti-inflammatory drugs (NSAIDs), are first prescribed. Corticosteroids may be prescribed for more serious illness, especially when tissue destruction is evident. In about fifteen percent of rheumatoid arthritis cases, these measures are ineffective, and stronger substances are used. Oral or injectable gold may prove helpful in treating rheumatoid arthritis. Some drugs usually used for cancer treatment may also be helpful.

Alternative physicians usually treat arthritis by recommending short fasts, screening for food allergies, recommending avoidance of processed foods, introducing fish and fish oils to the diet as well as anti-inflammatory herbal and nutritional supplements, and using natural methods to improve digestion. Alternative physicians may also recommend the substance glucosamine sulfate, which provides natural building blocks for cartilage, as a dietary supplement for those suffering from osteoarthritis. Scientific studies have suggested that supplementation with B vitamins, vitamin E, and some multiminerals (including the trace elements copper and selenium) may also improve the disease. On the other hand, studies have shown that nightshade vegetables—potatoes, tomatoes, bell peppers, and chili peppers—may provoke joint pain.

Very few of the herbs or foods recommended as a natural remedy for treating arthritis have been tested clinically for anti-inflammatory effects. Many of these herbs and foods contain plant constituents for which such effects are known, however.

Natural Remedies for Arthritis

Celery

The remedy of eating raw or cooked celery seeds (*Apium graveolens*) or large amounts of the celery plant to treat rheumatism arrived in North America with the British and German immigrants. Using celery to treat rheumatism persists today in North American professional herbalism. Various parts of the celery plant contain more than twenty-five different anti-inflammatory compounds. And, taken as a food, celery is rich in minerals: A cup of celery contains more than 340 milligrams of potassium. (A potassium deficiency may contribute to some symptoms of arthritis.)

You can place one teaspoon of celery seeds in a cup. Fill the cup with boiling water. Cover and let stand for fifteen minutes. Strain and drink three cups a day during any acute attacks.

Angelica

Angelica (*Angelica archangelica*), an herb that has been used in European folk medicine since antiquity, can be used to treat arthritis. The Western variety of angelica has twelve anti-inflammatory constituents, ten antispasmodic (muscle relaxant) constituents, and five anodyne (pain-relieving) ones. The Chinese sometimes use their native variety of the plant (*Angelica sinensis*) for the same purpose. The Chinese species is sold in North America under the names *dang gui* or *dong quai*.

You can place one tablespoon of the cut roots of either species of angelica in one pint of water and bring to a boil. Cover and boil for two minutes. Remove from heat and let stand, covered, until the water cools to room temperature. Strain and drink the tea in three doses during the day for two to three weeks at a time. Then, take a break for seven to ten days and start the treatment again if desired.

Rosemary

A collection of remedies by folklorist Clarence Meyer called *American Folk Medicine* suggests drinking rosemary tea to treat arthritis. The same remedy is used in the contemporary natural medicine of the Coahuila Indians in Mexico. Rosemary has not been tested in clinical trials, but it was used to successfully relieve pain by doctors of the Physiomedicalist school. The plant's leaves contain four anti-inflammatory substances—carnosol, oleanolic acid, rosmarinic acid, and ursolic acid.

Carnosol acts on the same anti-inflammatory pathways as both steroids and aspirin, oleanolic acid has been marketed as an antioxidant in China, rosmarinic acid acts as an anti-inflammatory, and ursolic acid, which makes up about four percent of the plant by weight, has been shown to have antiarthritic effects in animal trials.

Put 1/2 ounce of rosemary leaves in a one-quart canning jar and fill the jar with boiling water. Cover tightly and let stand for thirty minutes. Drink a cup of the hot tea before going to bed and have another cupful in the morning before breakfast. Do this for two to three weeks, and then take a break for seven to ten days before starting the treatment again.

Alfalfa

Alfalfa (*Medicago sativa*) is often promoted in health food stores as an arthritis remedy—in the form of capsulated alfalfa powder. Alfalfa contains L-canavanine, however, an amino acid that can cause symptoms that are similar to those of systemic lupus, an autoimmune disease that can also cause joint pain. Some scientific studies show that these symptoms can occur in both animals and humans as a result of eating alfalfa. Thus, the remedy below is best taken in the form of a tea rather than powder; the amino acid is not present to any significant amount in alfalfa tea. Alfalfa tea is rich with nutritive minerals. It is a recommended natural remedy for arthritis in southern Appalachia.

Place one ounce of alfalfa tea in a pot. Cover with one quart of water and boil for thirty minutes. Strain and drink the quart throughout the day. Do this for two to three weeks, and then take a break for seven to ten days before starting again.

Sesame Seeds

A remedy for arthritis from Chinese medicine is to eat sesame seeds. A half ounce of the seeds contains about 4 grams of essential fatty acids, 175 milligrams of calcium, 64 milligrams of magnesium, and, notably, .73 milligrams of copper. Increased copper intake may be important during arthritis attacks because the body's requirements go up during inflammation.

You can grind up 1/2 ounce of sesame seeds in a coffee grinder and sprinkle on your food at mealtime. You can use this treatment for as long as you like.

Headaches

A headache is a symptom of disease, and not a disease in itself. Rarely is a headache the symptom of a serious illness—most headaches are caused by minor conditions, such as muscle tension in the neck and around the skull or inflammation of blood vessels in the brain.

There are three basic types of headaches. The vascular headache occurs when blood vessels in the head enlarge and press on nerves, causing pain. The most common vascular headache is the migraine. The second type of headache is the muscle contraction headache, which results when the muscles of the face, neck, or scalp contract and tighten. A tension headache is an example

of a muscle contraction headache. The third kind of headache is the inflammatory headache. Such a headache is the result of pressure within the head. The causes range from relatively minor conditions, such as sinusitis, to more serious problems, such as brain tumors.

Headaches are most often treated with aspirin and nonsteroidal anti-inflammatory drugs (NSAIDs) such as ibuprofen or acetaminophen. Treatment of a migraine already in progress usually consists of a drug therapy program chosen from a variety of painkillers, sedatives, and special drugs and remedies, including vasoconstricting drugs and caffeine. Tension headaches can be treated by eliminating the tension or correcting the physical problem that is causing the headaches. This can sometimes be done through physical manipulation of the spine or skull by a chiropractic or osteopathic physician.

The herbal remedies for headaches, which are still used today by alternative physicians in the United States and by some conventional doctors in Europe, fall into four categories: pain relievers, anti-inflammatories, sedatives, and digestive herbs.

The pain-relieving and anti-inflammatory herbs may relieve most types of headaches. The sedatives work well for relieving tension headaches. The digestive herbs and laxatives are most useful for treating headaches that accompany digestive sluggishness or constipation.

Natural Remedies for Headaches

Willow Bark

More than 2,400 years ago, the Greeks used willow bark (*Salix* spp.) to treat headache pain. American Indians of the Alabama, Chickasaw, Houma, Montagnais, Shoshone, and Thompson tribes and the Ninivak Eskimos used it for the same purpose, even before the arrival of the European colonists.

Willow bark is still used to treat headache pain in the medicine of Indiana, New England, and the Southwest. It is recommended by professional medical herbalists of North America and Great Britain. The German government has approved its use by conventional physicians for treating pain and fever.

The most important active constituent in willow bark is salicin, but the bark also contains at least three other anti-inflammatory constituents. In Germany, the suggested dose is about one gram of the powdered bark—the amount in about two average-sized gelatin capsules. Willow bark is not as potent as aspirin, but it is less likely to cause stomach upset.

To make a tea, place two teaspoons of powdered willow bark in a cup and fill with boiling water. Let steep for fifteen to twenty minutes. Sweeten with honey as desired. Drink up to four cups a day. Note that salicin can cause skin rashes in some people.

Alternately, you can purchase willow bark capsules in a health food store or an herb shop. Take as directed on the product label.

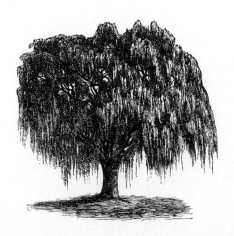

Rosemary-Sage Tea

A natural remedy for treating headache pain is to drink a tea of rosemary (*Rosmarinus officinalis*) and sage (*Salvia officinalis*). Rosemary has been a popular medicine in Europe for treating pain at least since the time of the ancient Greeks. Among the Greeks, rosemary had a reputation for improving memory.

Today, rosemary is used to soothe headaches in the traditional medicine of China, and, in the United States, it is used for the same purpose in Indiana and among the Amish. The German government has approved the use of rosemary for pain. There, rosemary is often used externally, in preparations such as salves and baths. It is a common folk use to apply rosemary to the temples in the form of a poultice to relieve headache pain.

Sage is not often used in natural medicine as a pain reliever, but it has an important chemical constituent in common with rosemary—rosmarinic acid. In addition, the combination of rosemary and sage contains more than twenty anti-inflammatory constituents, although some of these exist only in minute amounts. Seek medical attention for any headache that lasts longer than three days. Do not ingest rosemary in any amount exceeding those usually found in foods because of the herb's reputed abortifacient and emmenagogue effects.

To make a tea lace one teaspoon of crushed rosemary leaves and one teaspoon of crushed sage leaves in a cup. Fill with boiling water. Cover well to prevent the escape of volatile substances. Let steep until the tea reaches room temperature. Take 1/2-cup doses two or three times a day for two or three days. You don't have to mix rosemary and sage to find pain relief. You can also try drinking either rosemary or sage teas separately.

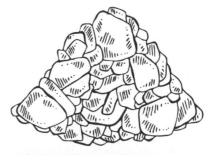

Yarrow

Yarrow (*Achillea millefolium*) has been used as a universal pain and headache remedy among various American Indian tribes, including the Cheyenne, Chippewa, Gosuite, Iroquois, Lummi, Mendocino, Navaho, Paiute, Seneca, and Shoshone. Yarrow contains anti-inflammatory constituents, including salicylic acid, an aspirin-like substance.

You can place one ounce of dried or fresh yarrow leaves in a one-quart jar and fill with boiling water. Cover tightly to prevent the escape of the aromatic constituents. The dose is one-half cup of the tea, two to four times a day. If any headache persists for more than three days, see your doctor.

Coffee or Tea

Coffee or tea is recommended as a headache cure in several traditions. Caffeine is the medicinal constituent responsible for the benefits. Caffeine is also used in conventional medicine to treat migraine headaches. It works by constricting the vessels of the brain, which are sometimes dilated during a headache attack. Tea is recommended in New England, and strong black coffee in Appalachia. Black coffee is a famous cure throughout Europe and North America for the type of headache that accompanies hangover.

You can make a pot of strong black coffee or tea and drink two cups to relieve an acute headache. Note that habitual use of caffeine can cause headache or withdrawal.

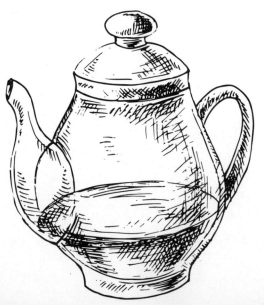

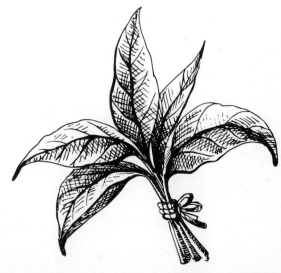

Mints

The mints—peppermint (*Mentha piperita*) and spearmint (*Mentha spicata*)—are used as headache remedies in the medicine of the particular regions where they are grown. American Indians of both eastern and western North America, including the Cherokee, Iroquois, Gosuite, and Paiute tribes, used these mints as headache remedies. Some tribes crushed the plant and inhaled the fumes; others placed the plant on the forehead or temples in the same way rosemary is used.

Today, mints are used in the medicine of China, Mexico, Appalachia, and the American Southwest to treat headaches. The mints contain about the same levels of the anti-inflammatory rosmarinic acid as do rosemary and sage.

You can place one ounce of dried mint leaves in a one-quart jar and fill with boiling water. Cover tightly to prevent the escape of the aromatic constituents. The dose is 1/2-cup of tea, two to four times a day. If a headache persists for more than three days, a visit to the doctor is in order.

Wormwood

Plants of the Artemisia genus (*Artemisia* spp.) have been used as pain remedies by at least twenty-two American Indian tribes throughout North America. Some tribes received the pain-relieving properties of the plants by burning them and inhaling their smoke and aromatic oils. To treat a headache, others made a tea of the leaves and used them as a wash on the forehead and temples. The use of the Artemisia species is recorded today in the natural medicine of northern New Mexico. The European species *Artemisia absinthum* (or wormwood) is approved as a digestive stimulant by the German government. Excessive use in large amounts can lead to brain damage, however.

The active constituents of plants in the Artemisia species include bitter digestive stimulants and anti-inflammatory volatile oils such as azulenes. These constituents are also present in yarrow and chamomile. You can place one teaspoon of wormwood leaves in a cup of water and fill with boiling water. Cover well. Let cool to room temperature. Take 1/2-cup doses every three hours for up to three days. If the headache persists, see a doctor.

Chapter 4:
Nature's Antibiotics

Probiotic Lifestyle and Gut Health

If the digestive tract is healthy and digestion and absorption of the nutrients are efficient, then the entire body will be well-nourished and will function optimally. Any irregularity in digestion, however, can cause or contribute to disease anywhere in the body.

Below are some common signs of a poorly functioning digestive system:

- flatulence or belching
- nausea
- pain anywhere in the digestive tract
- undigested food in the stool
- offensive breath
- constipation (less than one bowel movement per day)
- lethargy or depression after meals
- food cravings other than normal hunger
- lack of satisfaction after meals
- lack of hunger for breakfast

These symptoms—all considered to be serious signs that require treatment in traditional medical systems—are often left untreated by conventional physicians in North America. This is not so in the modern medicine of Germany and France, however, where symptoms such as "biliousness" (sluggish liver function), poor appetite, gas, and bloating, or feelings of fullness after meals, are routinely treated by doctors, often with herbal medicines from the European tradition.

According to natural medicine throughout the world, which offers many remedies for weak and sluggish digestion, healthy digestion requires:

- A balance of fats, proteins, and starches in the diet, and adequate fiber from sources such as grains, beans, fruits, and vegetables.
- A moderate intake of food quantities. Overeating strains the capacity of the digestive system to process the consumed food, and undigested or partially digested remnants can cause inflammation and other problems in the digestive tract and elsewhere in the body.

🦠 A relaxed state during meals. For the stomach and intestines to function normally, and for digestive secretions to be adequate, the body cannot be in a state of stress during meals.

🦠 A healthy number of normal bacteria in the gut.

The "garden" of friendly bacteria in the intestines acts as a defense against harmful bacteria, yeasts, molds, and other microorganisms by competing with them for food. (As the friendly bacteria proliferate, the nutrients they consume deprive the harmful micro organisms of their food supply.) Some of these friendly bacteria manufacture essential vitamins. The good bacteria can be disrupted by courses of such drugs as birth control pills, steroids, and antibiotics, however, leading to poor digestion and inflammation and infection of the intestinal wall. This in turn can cause inflammatory diseases in other parts of the body as the intestinal contents leak through the inflamed gut wall and overwhelm the immune system.

Natural remedies may improve digestion by stimulating the secretion of more stomach acid, digestive enzymes, and bile (a digestive secretion of the liver) from the liver. The remedies may also improve the absorption of nutrients by increasing blood flow to the mucous membranes of the intestines. Finally, antispasmodic constituents in some remedies may prevent spasms in intestinal wall muscles that often accompany gas and bloating. Any severe or persistent digestive tract symptoms merit a visit to your doctor.

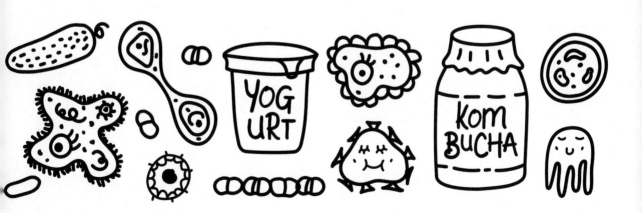

Factors That Affect Healthy Digestion

An intact and fully functional digestive tract provides the framework for healthy digestion and metabolism. Activity level, conditions and diseases, diet, genes, medications, stress, and other factors may affect healthy digestion.

Bacteria, fungi, and viruses are miniscule microbes that reside in the intestines as well as inside the genitalia, mouth, nose, urinary tract, and on the skin. A microbiome is a collection of these microbes that is unique for each individual. It is determined by genetics and lifestyle among other factors.

In the bigger picture, microbiome disruption and/or bacteria imbalances may be associated with conditions or diseases such as colon cancer, diabetes, and obesity. Microbiome bacteria imbalances may also contribute to inflammatory autoimmune diseases such as inflammatory bowel disease including Crohn's disease, lupus, and rheumatoid arthritis. Modifying one's microbiome through environmental and lifestyle changes may provide some insights into these diseases and others and outline courses of action.

Healthy Gut Flora

Since gut bacteria line the intestines, they are involved with the digestion and absorption of foods and beverages. Gut bacteria also help communicate with the body's immune system, influence brain functioning, and produce vitamins that are necessary for life.

It's possible that people with GI conditions and diseases have different compositions of gut bacteria that affect these functions and others. It may also be that a diversity of gut bacteria is more important than the presence or absence of specific gut bacteria.

Imbalanced gut bacteria may also be linked with attention-deficit-disorder, anxiety, autism, Alzheimer's disease, cardiovascular disease, and depression. This is because gut bacteria may be able to produce metabolites, or small molecules than may make their way to the brain, heart, and other organs and affect their normal functioning.

Improving Gut Flora

Gut flora may improve with a diet that is lower in fats and sugars and higher in certain fibers. By making certain dietary changes, a person may be able to alter their microbiome, improve their immune function, reduce inflammation, and be healthier overall. Drinking more water, managing stress, and incorporating exercise into daily activities may also help support a healthier microbiome.

Healthy gut bacteria may be increased through the addition of fermented foods with probiotics, live bacteria and yeasts that include certain types of yogurt, kefir (a yogurt-based beverage), miso, pickles, and sauerkraut. Another option is the use of probiotic supplements with similar functionality. Probiotic supplements are thought to be safe but they may have side effects and/or trigger allergic reactions.

People with depressed immune function due to chemotherapy or late-stage cancer should be cautioned about taking probiotic supplements since they may be incompatible with treatments.

To Increase Probiotics in Your Diet

Look for the following terms that generally indicate a product contains probiotics:

- Buttermilk
- Fermented milks
- Kefir
- Kim chi
- Miso
- Sauerkraut
- Some juice
- Some pickles
- Some soft cheese
- Some yogurt
- Soy drinks
- Tempeh

Dietary probiotics have various forms and functions, such as *acidophilus* (in yogurt and other fermented foods), *bifidobacterium* (in some dairy products such as some cheeses and yogurt), and *saccharomyces boulardii* (yeast found in some probiotic supplements). It is best to investigate what's right.

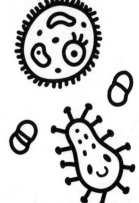

Natural Remedies for Digestion Problems

Natural remedies may improve digestion by stimulating the secretion of more stomach acid, digestive enzymes, and bile (a digestive secretion of the liver) from the liver. The remedies may also improve the absorption of nutrients by increasing blood flow to the mucous membranes of the intestines. Finally, antispasmodic constituents in some remedies may prevent spasms in intestinal wall muscles that often accompany gas and bloating. Remember, any severe or persistent digestive tract symptoms merit a visit to your doctor.

Ginger

Ginger (*Zingiber officinale*) is a remedy for treating gas or nausea in the traditions of both New England and the southern Appalachians. It is used the same way in the traditional medicine of India, China, and Arabia. Ginger contains at least thirteen antispasmodic constituents, which may help reduce spasms and tension in the digestive tract muscles. Also, circulatory stimulants in ginger increase circulation to the mucous membrane lining of the digestive tract, which in turn increases digestive secretions and absorption of nutrients. What's more, in clinical trials, ginger has shown to be effective in soothing some kinds of nausea and vertigo. Avoid excessive doses of ginger if you're taking drugs for heart or blood conditions or diabetes.

You can stir 1/2 teaspoon of ground ginger into a cup of hot water. Let stand two to three minutes. Strain and drink.

Mint

Different types of mints are recommended for treating indigestion in North American literature, most commonly peppermint (*Mentha piperita*) and spearmint (*Mentha spicata*). Mints appear in the medicine of New England, New York, Indiana, Appalachia, New Mexico, and California. Mints have also been used as carminatives by members of the Cherokee, Chippewa, Dakota, Omaha, Pawnee, Ponca, and Winnebago American Indian tribes. Mint species contain the antispasmodic constituents carvacrol, eugenol, limonene, and thymol, which may help reduce intestinal spasms. A contemporary German medical text, *Herbal Medicine* by R.F. Weiss, M.D., recommends the mints as digestive aids for their carminative and antispasmodic properties. Peppermint is used as an official digestive aid in Germany.

Place one teaspoon of the dried herb in a cup and add boiling water. Cover and let stand for ten minutes. Strain well and drink the tea warm three times a day on an empty stomach. Don't use peppermint if you are experiencing heartburn or painful belches.

Fennel

A tea of fennel seeds (*Foeniculum vulgare*) is used for treating sluggish digestion or gas in the medicine of both New England and China. It is also the most often prescribed tea for abdominal cramping and gas in adults in the medical herbalism of contemporary Great Britain, Canada, and the United States. It is an approved medicine in Germany for mild gastrointestinal complaints. At least sixteen

chemical constituents in fennel have demonstrated antispasmodic effects in animal trials.

You can place one teaspoon of the seeds in a cup and add boiling water. Cover and let stand for ten minutes. Strain and drink three cups of warm tea a day on an empty stomach until digestion improves.

Caraway Seeds

Caraway seeds (*Carum carvi*), with a flavor and a medicinal action similar to that of fennel, are recommended for gas and poor digestion in Appalachia and in the medicine of Indiana. Their medicinal use originated in Arab culture. Their use for poor digestion spread to ancient Rome, and from there to European medicine. Caraway seeds are approved for medical use for weak digestion by the German government.

In a cup, pour boiling water over one teaspoon of the crushed seeds. Cover and let stand for ten minutes. Strain well and drink three cups of warm tea a day on an empty stomach. Alternately, you can chew on the seeds. A common practice in households in India and the Middle East is to pass a small bowl of caraway, fennel, or anise seeds for nibbling after meals.

Garlic Battles Infections

Garlic's potential to combat heart disease has received a lot of attention, but it should receive even more acclaim for its antimicrobial properties. Fresh, raw garlic has proven itself since ancient times as an effective killer of bacteria and viruses.

Laboratory studies confirm that raw garlic has antibacterial and antiviral properties. Not only does it knock out many common cold and flu viruses, but its effectiveness also spans a broad range of both gram-positive and gram-negative bacteria (two major classifications of bacteria), fungus, intestinal parasites, and yeast. Cooking garlic, however, destroys the allicin, so you'll need to use raw garlic to prevent or fight infections.

Antimicrobial Activity

Garlic's infection-fighting capability was confirmed in a study conducted by researchers at the University of Ottawa that was published in the April 2005 issue of *Phytotherapy Research*. Researchers tested 19 natural health products that contain garlic and five fresh garlic extracts for active compounds and antimicrobial activity. They tested the effectiveness of these substances against three types of common bacteria: *E. faecalis*, which causes urinary tract infections; *N. gonorrhoeae*, which causes the sexually transmitted disease gonorrhea; and *S. aureus*, which is responsible for many types of infections that are common in hospitals.

The products most successful at eradicating these bacteria were the ones with the highest allicin content. Now garlic is being investigated to see whether it can help us battle microbes that are resistant to antibiotics. One simple but meaningful demonstration of garlic's antibacterial power can be found in a study conducted at the University of California, Irvine. Garlic juice was tested in the laboratory against a wide spectrum of potential pathogens, including several antibiotic-resistant strains of bacteria. It showed significant activity against the pathogens. Even more exciting was the fact that garlic juice still retained significant antimicrobial activity, even in dilutions ranging up to 1:128 of the original juice.

Is it possible that garlic can work alongside prescription medications to both reduce side effects and to help the drugs work better? Results from several studies say yes. In a Rutgers University study that used bacteria in lab dishes, garlic and two common antibiotics were pitted against certain antibiotic-resistant strains of *S. aureus* (a grampositive bacteria) and *E. coli* (a gram-negative bacteria).

Garlic was able to significantly increase the effectiveness of the two antibiotic medications in killing the bacteria. Research done in Mexico City at a facility supported by the National Institutes of Health of Mexico also showed some interesting results. It extended previous research in rats that used aged garlic extract and various sulfur-containing compounds from garlic along with gentamicin, a powerful antibiotic that can cause kidney damage. When any of the garlic compounds was ingested along with gentamicin, kidney damage was diminished.

Next, researchers set about to determine whether garlic weakened the effectiveness of genta-

micin. As it turns out, the exact opposite happened: Garlic actually enhanced the effect of gentamicin. These findings indicate that with the use of garlic, perhaps less gentamicin would be needed, and kidney damage could be minimized.

Judging by research conducted in lab dishes and animals, it appears that garlic is a strong defender against microbes, even against those that have developed a resistance to common antibiotics. It also appears that garlic enhances the effects of some traditional antibiotics. But does it stand up to the test in humans?

Battling the Bugs Within

Eating raw garlic may help combat the sickness-causing bugs that get loose inside our bodies. Garlic has been used internally as a folk remedy for years, but now the plant is being put to the test scientifically for such uses. So far, its grades are quite good as researchers pit it against a variety of bacteria.

For eons, herbalists loaded soups and other foods with garlic and placed garlic compresses on people's chests to provide relief from colds and chest congestion. Now the Mayo Clinic has stated, "Preliminary reports suggest that garlic may reduce the severity of upper respiratory tract infection." The findings have not yet passed the scrutiny of numerous, large, well-designed human studies, so current results are classified as "unclear."

Can a garlic clove help stop your sniffles? A study published in the July/August 2001 issue of *Advances in Therapy* examined the stinking rose's ability to fight the common cold. The study involved 146 volunteers divided into two groups. One group took a garlic supplement for 12 weeks during the winter months, while the other group received a placebo. The group that received garlic had significantly fewer colds—and the colds that they did get went away faster—than the placebo group.

Garlic also may help rid the intestinal tract of Giardia lamblia, a parasite that commonly lives in stream water and causes giardiasis, an infection of the small intestine. Hikers and campers run the risk of this infection whenever they drink untreated stream or lake water. Herbalists prescribe a solution of one or more crushed garlic cloves stirred into one-third of a cup of water taken three times a day to eradicate Giardia. If you're fighting giardiasis, be sure to consult your health-care provider, because it's a

nasty infection. Ask if you can try garlic as part of your treatment.

Finally, in the January 2005 issue of *Antimicrobial Agents and Chemotherapy*, researchers reported the results of an investigation into whether fresh garlic extract would inhibit *C. albicans*, a cause of yeast infections. The extract was very effective in the first hour of exposure to *C. albicans*, but the effectiveness decreased during the 48-hour period it was measured. However, conventional antifungal medications have the same declining effectiveness as time passes.

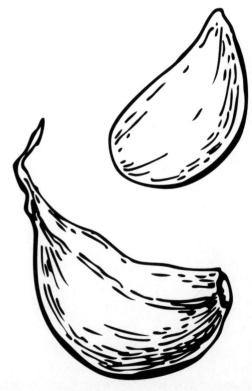

Remedies for a Sore Throat

A bacterial infection or lots of singing, talking, or yelling can cause a sore throat. At times, the throat can be so inflamed and painful that it becomes difficult to swallow. If the inflammation is in the voice box, you can easily come down with laryngitis, in which your voice is reduced to a hoarse whisper or it even may become impossible to talk at all. For centuries, European singers have known the secret to preserving their voices with aromatherapy and herbal remedies. Their most popular sore throat and laryngitis cure is to gargle with a marjoram herb tea that has been sweetened with honey. You can use the essential oil of marjoram to make a similar remedy. As both an antiseptic and anti-inflammatory, it is a good choice. Other essential oils or herb teas to use as a gargle are sage, hyssop, and thyme, all of which kill bacterial infections.

Any of these essential oils can easily be gargled or sprayed into the throat. This brings the anti-bacterial and soothing essential oils into direct contact with the bacteria responsible for causing a sore throat or laryngitis. In an emergency, a few drops of essential oil diluted in two ounces of water may also be used. Both lavender and eucalyptus work so well in an aromatherapy steam to recover your voice that you must remind yourself to not overstress it until your throat fully recovers. And don't forget the old standard of a hot drink made with fresh lemon juice and honey. Essential oils for sore throat: bergamot, eucalyptus, lavender, lemon, marjoram, sage, sandalwood, tea tree, thyme.

Throat Spray

You will need:

- 4 drops marjoram oil
- ½ cup warm water
- ¼ teaspoon salt

Combine ingredients. Shake well to dissolve the salt and disperse the oils before spraying or gargling. Gargle every half hour at first and then several times a day.

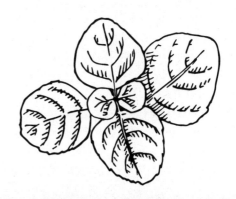

Remedies for Congestion

The most common cause of sinus and lung congestion is a cold or flu virus. Additionally, secondary bacterial infections that follow on the heels of colds and flus can be especially nasty, irritating the delicate lining in the respiratory tract. The mucous that causes the congestion is produced to protect that lining and wash away the infection.

For quick relief, thin out congestion by using the essential oils of eucalyptus, peppermint, and bergamot combined with steam. Remember how much easier it is to breath when you step into a steamy, hot shower? The steam opens up tightened bronchial passages, allowing the essential oils to penetrate and wipe out the viral or bacterial infection that is causing the problem.

Two of the best essential oils to eliminate infection are lavender and eucalyptus. In fact, studies prove that a two percent dilution of eucalyptus oil kills 70 percent of airborne *staphylococcus* bacteria. Anise, peppermint, and eucalyptus reduce coughing, perhaps by suppressing the brain's cough reflex. If conges-

tion is severe, also use essential oils that loosen congestion. Cypress dries a persistently runny nose.

To create a therapeutic steam, add a few drops of essential oil to a pan of water that is simmering on the stove. You can also use a humidifier—some actually provide a compartment for essential oils. If you are at the office or traveling and steaming is impractical, try inhaling a tissue scented with the oils, or use a natural nasal inhaler.

Vapor Rub

You will need:

- 12 drops eucalyptus oil
- 5 drops peppermint oil
- 5 drops thyme oil
- 1 ounce olive oil

Combine ingredients in a glass bottle. Shake well to mix oils evenly. Gently massage into chest and throat. Use one to five times per day and especially just before bed.

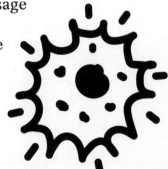

Germ Fighter Spray

You will need:

- 12 drops tea tree oil
- 6 drops eucalyptus oil
- 6 drops lemon oil
- 2 ounces distilled water

Combine the ingredients, and shake well to disperse the oils before each use. Dispense this formula from a spray bottle on minor cuts, burns, or abrasions to prevent infection and speed healing. As an alternative to distilled water, you can use a tincture made from an antiseptic herb such as Oregon grape root. Keep in mind that tinctures contain alcohol, which will make the essential oils disperse better and increase the antiseptic properties of the spray, but it will also sting more on an open wound. Apply immediately and then several times a day to keep the wound clean and encourage healing.

Remedies for Bladder Infections

Bladder infections are common, especially in women. So common, in fact, that you may already be familiar with the medical term cystitis to describe the inflammation that can result when bladder infections are unattended.

Fortunately, several essential oils can come to the rescue. Juniper berry, sandalwood, chamomile, pine, tea tree, and bergamot are especially effective treatments. However, juniper berry is so strong that it could irritate the kidneys if the bladder infection has spread into them. If that is the case, stick to the other oils. In fact, if there is any chance that you have a kidney infection, be sure to seek a doctor's opinion, as it can have serious consequences.

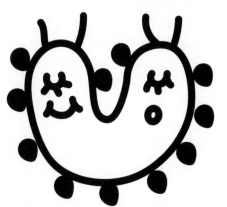

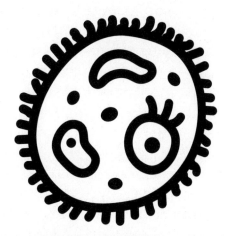

Bladder Infection Oil

You will need:

- 8 drops juniper berry or cypress oil
- 6 drops tea tree oil
- 6 drops bergamot oil
- 2 drops fennel oil
- 2 ounces vegetable oil

Combine the ingredients. Massage over the bladder area once daily. For a preventive treatment, add a tablespoon of this same oil to your bath.

Cold and Flu

A simple common cold is a collection of familiar symptoms signaling an infection of the upper respiratory tract, which includes the nose, throat, and sinuses. At least five major categories of viruses cause colds. One of these groups, and perhaps the most common, the rhinoviruses, includes a minimum of 100 different viruses. The viruses that cause a cold reproduce in the mucous membranes. The viruses do not penetrate deeper into the body—into the gastrointestinal tract, for example—because they cannot survive at the higher body temperatures there.

Although we often say "colds and flu" in the same breath, influenza is a very different disease from the common cold. The influenza virus takes up residence mainly in the throat and bronchial tract. If you have the flu, you usually have a fever, and a fever is not usually present in a cold. The fever usually passes within three days, but the fatigue, muscle aches, and cough that result from the flu can linger for weeks. Influenza will not seriously injure a normally healthy person, but those with preexisting lung conditions, the elderly, and others with weakened resistance are especially prone to the flu's deadly effects.

Flu is known as the "Last of the Great Plagues" because it kills so many people worldwide each year, including about 20,000 Americans. And when highly virulent flu strains periodically erupt, the death toll can rise even higher. For example, a flu epidemic just after World War I killed more than 30 million people worldwide.

The conventional treatment for flu in those at high risk for fatal complications is immunization in late fall with a flu vaccine. Immunization is also recommended for those who care for such high-risk patients. The antiviral drug ribavarin can be taken as well; it may be effective in preventing severe pneumonia caused by the influenza virus. Some patients request antibiotics from their doctors to treat a cold or flu episode, and unfortunately, many doctors comply. Antibiotic drugs are good only for bacterial infections and are ineffective against colds and flu. In fact, taking them inappropriately may promote the development of drug-resistant bacterial strains and may render the antibiotics ineffective later on when the patient really needs them. The drug resistant strains can also be passed on to others.

Aspirin and other pain-killing drugs are also inappropriate treatments for cold and flu. Even though they may provide some temporary relief, they may suppress the immune system and can actually prolong the infection. And giving aspirin to children for colds and flu is a no-no. In rare cases, it can lead to the development of Reye syndrome, a serious and often fatal neurological disorder.

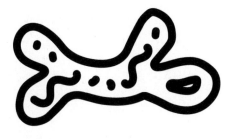

Remedies for the Cold and Flu

Echinacea

Echinacea (*Echinacea angustifolia, Echinacea purpurea*) is, without a doubt, the most commonly used natural remedy for treating colds and flu in the United States today. In fact, echinacea is the best-selling medicinal herb in the country.

Echinacea was used as a remedy by the American Indians of the Great Plains states. The tribes residing in those areas used the herb for all manner of infectious diseases. Eclectic physicians, a now-defunct North American school of doctors who used herbs as medicines, adopted the use of echinacea in the mid-1880s. By 1920, it was the remedy they prescribed the most. The use of echinacea spread to Germany in the 1930s, where it remains an approved medicine today—used to treat colds, flu, and other conditions related to underlying deficiencies of the immune system.

Echinacea is also famous in the contemporary medical herbalism of Britain, Australia, and North America for its ability to "abort" a cold or flu. German clinical trials show that echinacea, taken preventively during cold and flu season, can reduce the frequency and severity of a viral infection. In fact, if echinacea is taken at the first onset of symptoms, the cold may never develop at all. Once a cold has set in, however, the other remedies in the section may be more beneficial.

Purchase a tincture of echinacea at a health food store, herb shop, or drugstore. At the first sign of a cold or flu, take one teaspoon of the tincture every hour for three hours. If the infection persists, take one dropperful every three hours.

Elder Flower

Elderberry comprises about thirteen species of deciduous shrubs native to North America and Europe. European settlers brought elderberry plants with them to the American colonies. The Paiute and Shoshone Indians in the Rocky Mountain region used the leaves and flowers of a North American species of elderberry to treat colds, flu, and fevers.

A tea made of elderberry flowers is approved by the German government as a medicine for colds, especially if a cough is present. The flower tea is also used to treat colds and flu in the natural medicine of contemporary Indiana. The Michigan Amish use the tea as well.

Recent research in Israel and Panama has shown that elderberry juice stimulates the immune system and also directly inhibits the influenza virus. Constituents in the plant's flowers and berries seem to have immunosuppressant properties that help inactivate the influenza virus, halting its spread. Elderberry has been shown to be effective against eight different strains of the flu virus.

Drinking too much elderberry tea, more than indicated in the directions below, however, can leave you feeling nauseous. And, because of a documented diuretic effect, prolonged use may result in hypokalemia, or potassium loss. Avoid the use of elder during pregnancy and lactation.

You can place 1/2 ounce of elderberry flowers in a one quart canning jar and fill with boiling water. Cover and let steep for twenty minutes. Strain and pour a cup of the tea. Sweeten with honey. Take one cup once every four hours when you have a cold or flu. Wrap yourself up in warm blankets after drinking the tea to help induce sweating.

Yarrow

The ancient Greeks used yarrow (*Achillea millefolium*) as a remedy for colds, flu, and fever. At least eighteen American Indian tribes from all corners of North America used yarrow for the same purpose. The early colonists throughout North America used yarrow as a household medicine for a wide variety of ailments, usually conditions that were infectious or inflammatory in nature. The use of yarrow tea for colds and flu survives today in the medicine of North Carolina, Indiana, and upstate New York. Yarrow has documented anti-inflammatory, antispasmodic, diuretic, mild sedative, and moderate antibacterial activities.

You can place one ounce of dried or fresh yarrow in a one-quart canning jar. Fill the jar with boiling water and cover tightly. Let steep for twenty minutes. Strain, pour, and sweeten with honey. Take three cups a day, bundling up in blankets and resting in bed after each cup.

Ginger

Ginger tea is a cold remedy mentioned in the literature of New England, Appalachia, North Carolina, Indiana, and even China. Ginger induces sweating, which helps to cool the body during fever. Ginger contains twelve different aromatic anti-inflammatory compounds, including some with aspirin-like effects. Its other proven actions result from its anti-nausea and antivertigo properties. Ginger also has carminative (gas relieving), diaphoretic (sweat inducing), and antispasmodic activities.

Cut a fresh ginger root into thin slices (about the size of your thumb) and place in a pot with one quart of water. Bring to a boil, then cover the pot and simmer on the lowest possible heat for 30 minutes. Let cool for 30 minutes more before straining. Strain and drink 1/2 to one cup three to five times a day. Sweeten with honey, as desired (but never give honey to a child younger than two).

Peppermint

Peppermint (*Mentha piperita*) is a natural remedy used in Indiana to treat colds. Cornmint (*Mentha arvensis*), a close relative of the plant, is used in China for the same purpose. Both plants, when taken as a hot tea, induce sweating and help to cool a fever. Also, the essential oils in the plants, including menthol, act as decongestants when drunk as a tea or inhaled. Peppermint also has antispasmodic and carminative properties.

You can place 1/2 ounce of peppermint leaves in a one-quart jar. Fill the jar with boiling water and cover tightly. Let steep twenty minutes. Strain the liquid and drink two or three cups a day. Wrap yourself in blankets and rest in bed after each cup.

Horsemint-Beebalm Tea

Two closely related species, horsemint (*Monarda punctata*) and beebalm (*Monarda menthaefolia, M. didyma*), are used in natural medicine similarly to the way thyme is used. (Horsemint is native to the eastern United States; beebalm to the Rocky Mountains.) Both plants, like thyme, contain high amounts of the constituent thymol, which acts as an expectorant and antiseptic. Both plants also induce sweating and can help cool a fever.

You can put one teaspoon of dried leaves of either plant in a cup and fill with boiling water. Let steep for five minutes while inhaling

the fumes through both the nose and mouth. Strain, sweeten with honey, and sip the tea slowly. Do this three to five times a day.

Thyme

Thyme tea (*Thymus vulgaris*) is recommended as a treatment for cold or flu in the natural medicine of Indiana and China. Thyme taken in the form of a hot tea also induces sweating and helps to cool a fever. In addition, its constituent oil, thymol, is a powerful expectorant and antiseptic. The constituent readily disperses in the steam of a hot tea. Inhaling the steam may effectively spread the thymol throughout the mucous membranes of the upper respiratory tract and bronchial tree.

Thus, thymol may help inhibit bacteria, viruses, or fungi from infecting the membranes. Thyme also has mild analgesic and antipyretic(fever reducing) properties. This remedy from Indiana suggests sipping the tea slowly while inhaling its fragrance. In China, the same method is used as a preventive—for when colds or flu are "going around."

Put one teaspoon of dried thyme leaves in a cup and fill with boiling water. Let steep for five minutes while inhaling the fumes through both the nose and mouth. Then, strain the tea, sweeten with honey, and sip slowly. Go to bed and bundle up warmly in blankets.

Lemon Balm

Several Indiana residents responding to a poll of natural remedies in the 1980s recommended lemon balm (*Melissa officinalis*) tea for cold and flu. The plant, which is native to southern Europe and northern Africa, now grows throughout North America as well. Lemon balm has long been used as a relaxing and sweat inducing herb. The 12th century German mystic and healer Hildegarde von Bingen stated, "Lemon balm contains within it the virtues of a dozen other plants."

Lemon balm is approved today by the German government as a medicine for digestive complaints and sleeping disorders, though it is not recommended specifically for colds or flu. Its aromatic oils contain anti-viral compounds that may help disinfect the mucous membranes, however. Of the sweat-inducing herbs included in this section, lemon balm is probably the mildest and the most suitable for use in children. Lemon balm is also a mild sedative and can help relax a restless patient suffering from cold or flu.

You can place one teaspoon of the dried herb in a cup and fill with boiling water. Let steep for ten minutes. Inhale the steam from the cup. Strain and drink up to four cups a day. Sweeten with honey as desired.

Garlic

The recommendation to take garlic for colds comes from New England, the American Southwest, and all the way from China. Garlic has been used for colds, bronchial problems, and fevers in cultures throughout the world since the dawn of written medical history—even the ancient Egyptians used it to treat cough and fever.

Garlic's constituents are antibacterial, antiviral, and antifungal. Garlic also stimulates the immune system, increasing the body's resistance to invaders. In addition, garlic is an expectorant and induces sweating, helping to reduce fever. Garlic has been approved as a medicine for colds and coughs and a variety of other illnesses by the pharmaceutical regulatory commission of the European Union, a confederation of modern European nations that has dropped trade barriers and is working toward economic regulation and a common currency. Garlic can also lower cholesterol and thin the blood. Note that garlic taken in high doses can irritate the stomach.

You can blend three cloves of garlic in a blender with a little water. (A clove must be cut or crushed in order to release its constituents.) If you want, add half a lemon, skin and all, to the garlic. Put the contents in a cup and fill the cup with boiling water. Let steep for five minutes, inhaling the fragrance. Strain, add honey, and drink the entire cup in sips.

Do this two to three times a day while you have a cold or flu or once a day to prevent infection during epidemics. Alternately, peel and chop three whole garlic bulbs and soak them in one pint of wine (red or white) in a closed container for a month. Shake the jar once a day. Then, strain and take one tablespoon of the wine each day as a preventive measure.

Onion

Onions are used to treat colds in virtually every folk tradition in North America—whether eaten raw, roasted, or boiled; taken in the form of teas, milk, or wine; worn in a sock or in a bag around the neck; or applied to the chest as a poultice. Wild onions have been used for the same purpose by American Indian tribes in every region of the country. Using onions to treat colds continues today in the natural medicine of New England, upstate New York, North Carolina, Appalachia, Indiana, and within Chinese cultures throughout North America.

The constituents in onions—the same that cause onion's volatile vapors to burn the eyes—are antimicrobial. Onions also have expectorant qualities, which induce the flow of healthy cleansing mucous. Onions induce sweating as well.

You can cut up one whole large onion and simmer in a covered pot for twenty minutes. Strain if desired to remove pulp. Drink a cup of the tea three to four times daily when you have a cold or flu. Alternately, try chewing raw onions—but don't swallow until the onions are thoroughly chewed.

Sage

Some residents of New England, North Carolina, and Indiana recommend hot sage tea to "break up" a cold. Sage (*Salvia officinalis*) contains volatile oils, which have been shown to kill viruses in laboratory studies. It specifically kills the rhinovirus, the virus most often responsible for causing colds. Also, because of sage's astringent qualities, it traditionally was used to treat sore throats. So, if you are suffering a sore throat with your cold, hot sage tea may be just the remedy for you. Other documented properties of sage include mild hypotensive effects, anti-inflammatory properties, and analgesic and anticonvulsant effects.

You can place one teaspoon of sage in a cup and fill with boiling water. Cover and let steep for ten minutes. Strain, add a little lemon and honey, and drink. Repeat three to four times a day for as long as you have a cold.

Vinegar

A cold remedy from Indiana calls for inhaling the fumes of vinegar. This remedy is as old as ancient Greece—the Greek physician Hippocrates recommended the treatment for coughs and respiratory infections. Vinegar is a weak acid. Inhaling its fumes changes the acidity of the mucous membranes in the upper respiratory tract, making the membranes inhospitable to viruses. Due to its acidic nature, avoid splashing vinegar into the eyes or onto cuts.

In a jar, pour 1/2 cup of boiling water over 1/2 cup of vinegar. Gently inhale the steam. Be careful not to burn yourself.

Lemon

The contemporary natural remedies of New England and Indiana call for drinking "hot lemonade" during a cold or flu. The practice is at least as old as the ancient Romans. Lemon juice, like vinegar, is acidic. Drinking it helps to acidify the mucous membranes, making the membranes inhospitable to bacteria or viruses. Lemon oil, which gives the juice its fragrance, is like a pharmacy in itself—it contains antibacterial, antiviral, antifungal, and anti-inflammatory constituents. Five of the constituents are specifically active against the influenza virus. Lemon oil is also an expectorant, increasing the flow of healthy mucous. And lemon is very tasty—its flavor is used to promote compliance in taking cold and flu products.

You can place one chopped whole lemon—skin, pulp, and all—in a pot and add one cup of boiling water. While letting the mixture steep for five minutes, inhale the fumes. Then, strain and drink. Do this at the onset of a cold, and repeat three to four times a day for the duration of the cold.

Healing the Skin

The reason why treatments for skin conditions are so plentiful is because skin ailments, although usually minor as far as health risk is concerned, are so common. But skin conditions are also visible and uncomfortable and demand our attention.

Over time, useless natural remedies for the skin were smoothly weeded out—many were topical remedies, so it was usually obvious whether they worked or not. People kept the skin remedies that worked effectively and incorporated them into tradition.

In this chapter, we'll discuss remedies for heat rash, chapped skin, burns, and remedies designed for better overall health of the skin. Any infection of the skin that develops red streaks around it requires immediate medical attention.

Scarred for Life?

Reduction or elimination of scars is a common human desire, and remedies to reduce scarring appear in several North American traditions. Scars result from wound healing or from inflammation. This natural process leaves the injured tissue stronger than it was before the injury. Most agents that suppress scar formation, herbal or not, also tend to suppress healing. Treatments must be applied as soon as the wound is closed. Coconut oil, cocoa butter, castor oil, and vitamin E oil are all used as natural remedies.

Herbs Used for Skin Care

Red Clover

Red clover (*Trifolium pratense*) is a commonly used remedy for treating skin conditions (such as acne, eczema, boils, and rashes). It can be applied externally, which is recorded in the traditions of Indiana, or it can be taken as a tea, which is the practice in the southern Appalachian region.

Red clover tea is also one of the most often prescribed remedies for skin conditions in professional medical herbalism in North America. Red clover was used both internally and externally for skin conditions by the Eclectic physicians at the turn of the century. Harvey Felter, M.D., an Eclectic professor of medicine, said in his *King's American Dispensatory* that red clover, when applied externally, soothes inflamed skin, disinfects it, and promotes the growth of healthy tissue.

The plant contains more than thirty identified chemical constituents. Besides containing antimicrobial and anti-inflammatory chemicals, red clover also contains allantoin, which promotes the healing and growth of healthy skin tissue.

For external use, try this remedy from Indiana: Simmer whole flowering red clover plants until tender. Use just enough water to cover. Strain, press the plants into a thick mass, and sprinkle with white flour. (The flour helps add consistency to the poultice.) Place the floured poultice directly on the irritated skin. Leave on for about half an hour. You can use the red clover poultice several times a day. (The poultice can last a few days if it's kept in the refrigerator between applications.) The poultice is designed to help reduce inflammation and promote healing.

Jojoba Oil

The Papago Indian tribe of the Southwest has used jojoba nut (*Simmondsia chinensis*) preparations to treat skin conditions such as boils and rashes. The nuts are traditionally dried and then pulverized and applied to the skin. Jojoba oil is now commercially extracted, and it is a popular addition to skin creams, oils, and ointments available in health food stores. The oil is also used today in the traditional medicine of the Southwest for chapped skin. To soothe your chapped skin, you can apply commercial jojoba oil as desired.

Plantain Leaves

Plantain leaves (*Plantago major*) are a common weed found on lawns throughout the United States. It was naturalized in North America after the arrival of the Europeans. American Indians called it "White Man's Footprint" because it seemed to follow the European colonists wherever they went. The Delaware, Mohegan, Ojibwa, Cherokee, and other American Indian tribes used plantain for treating minor wounds and insect bites.

Plantain has been used in cultures around the world to treat wounds and skin conditions. Plantain contains a pharmacy of constituents that are beneficial to the skin, including at least fifteen anti-inflammatory constituents and six analgesic chemicals. Like red clover, it contains the constituent allantoin, which promotes cell proliferation and tissue healing. You can crush a small handful of fresh plantain leaves and apply the juice locally to dry, chapped skin.

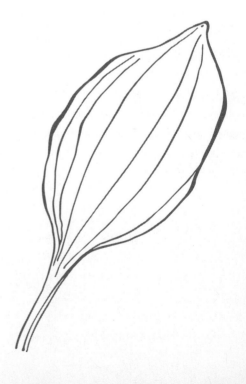

Oatmeal

Oatmeal is also a treatment for chapped hands per folklorist Clarence Meyer. In the method described below, oatmeal is used to both moisten and dry the skin. To treat chapped hands with oatmeal use wet oatmeal instead of soap to wash chapped hands. Then, after drying hands with a towel, rub the hands with dry oatmeal.

Clay

Clay application is a common natural remedy for treating various skin conditions throughout the world. It was common among the North American Indians even before the arrival of the European colonists. Today, the therapeutic use of clay makes up an important part of modern Seventh Day Adventist traditions. Clay is drawing and cooling. It is most effective on moist and inflamed conditions rather than on dry, chapped skin.

For a remedy purchase bentonite clay or cosmetic grade clay at a health food store or drugstore. Mix the clay with water to make a paste and apply to the skin. Allow to dry, then gently flake off after a few hours. Wipe the clay off over a bowl. Discard the waste in your garden or on your lawn, because clay can stop up your pipes. Apply clay every few hours.

Cornstarch & Cornmeal

Cornstarch and cornmeal are common agents used to treat moist skin conditions such as heat rash. They are also used to heal chapped skin and prickly heat. Cornstarch "dusting powder" appears in the contemporary folklore of Indiana. You can wash the affected area, wipe it dry, and dust with cornstarch.

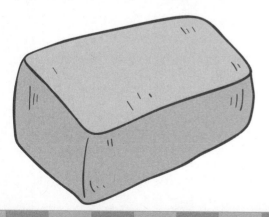

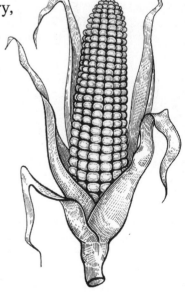

Rosemary

Rosemary leaf (*Rosmarinus officinalis*) is a remedy from the Southwest for treating windburn and cracked and chapped skin. It is also used in that region (and other areas as well) as a wash for infectious skin conditions. The plant's leaf contains four anti-inflammatory substances—carnosol, oleanolic acid, rosmarinic acid, and ursolic acid. Rosemary also contains more than ten antiseptic constituents.

To prepare you can crush rosemary leaves and warm in a pan on low heat. Add some lard to make a salve. Simmer over low heat until the lard takes on the color and aroma of the rosemary. Let cool. Apply to the affected areas as desired.

Vitamin E Oil

Vitamin E oil rubbed into scar tissue will help to reduce a scar, according to the traditions of the Amish. The Amish also use cocoa butter and castor oil for the same purpose. All three oils contain vitamin E, but the vitamin E oil contains higher amounts. Vitamin E has been shown to reduce scarring in a variety of scientific experiments. Treatment with vitamin E for skin grafts after severe burns did not work in one trial, however, so there may be a limit as to what can be accomplished with this simple remedy.

As soon as possible after a wound is closed, rub vitamin E oil (or one of the other oils above) into the tissues for five to ten minutes twice a day. The rubbing, which increases circulation and can break up deep scars, is an important part of the application process. Continue rubbing in the oil on a daily basis for months if necessary, or at least until improvement appears.

Potato Poultice

According to medical traditions of the Romani, a potato poultice will improve puffy skin, especially those "bags" under the eyes. This same method is taught in contemporary naturopathic medical schools to reduce inflammation of the skin. To make a poultice, thoroughly clean two or three potatoes. Grate (including the potato skins) and press them with your hands into a paste. Apply to the affected areas of the skin. Leave in place while relaxing for fifteen minutes. Remove the poultice and clean and dry the area.

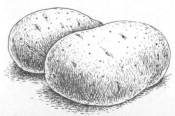

Fighting Aging

Taking care of your skin throughout your life is one of the best ways to prevent your face from advertising your years. Moisturizing your skin and protecting it from sunburns is essential for your skin to remain vibrant throughout old age. Below we will address how coconut oil can help restore your skin and how you can naturally heal from sunburns you may incur.

Coconuts, Sun Damage, and Aging

Sun damage occurs due to sun exposure throughout the years from everyday activities, as well as from conscious sunbathing. The changes in the earth's ozone layer are also responsible for undesirable ultraviolet (UV) radiation. Fair-skinned and darker-skinned individuals are both prone to sun damage; however, fairer-skinned individuals are more at risk.

In some parts of the world where there is intense and non-stop sun exposure, residents do not seem to have the same type of sun damage that they do in other locations. It may be that their local diets are more abundant in antioxidant–rich foods and vegetables that feed and protect the skin from the inside out.

Cellular degeneration may be caused by free radicals in the environment. Free radicals may be formed as the result of exposure to sunlight and air pollutants, but they may also be due to alcohol consumption, diet, drugs, exercise, inflammation, smoking, and one's diet.

One method to delay or prevent cellular degeneration from free radicals is with a diet that is rich in antioxidants (substances that help to halt oxidation which causes cellular destruction). Coconut oil has some antioxidants, but it is more valuable for its saturated fatty acids. A diet that is high in polyunsaturated fatty acids may lead to cellular membrane instability and make one more prone to cellular damage by the sun and environmental factors. Saturated fats are more protective.

Coconut oil, when liberally applied to the skin, also helps to retain the skin's moisture and shiny appearance in hot, dry conditions and promotes all-over tanning, if desired. Aging affects the skin since it loses hydration and flexibility and the healing process takes longer than in younger skin. When coupled with the constant exposure to ultraviolet radiation and increased damage by free radicals, aging skin may look dry, old, saggy, and wrinkly. Coconut oil to the rescue!

Coconut oil may be used to treat weathered skin or even to help guard against the grim ravages of ultraviolet radiation. However, coconut oil may not be a cure-all for advanced skin problems. Before using, check with a specialist for prescribed care.

Remedies for Burns and Sunburns

Vinegar: Vinegar washes are recommended in natural remedies from New England and New Mexico. Vinegar is both an astringent and antiseptic, and like cool water, it helps to prevent blisters. You can apply vinegar to a burn every few minutes. Dilute the vinegar if the skin is very sensitive.

Tobacco: An American Indian treatment for burns is to wash the area in tobacco tea. Indiana medical folklore suggests applying a wad of chewing tobacco to the burned area. You can remove the tobacco from a package of cigarettes and add it to one quart of water. Boil the water until the volume is reduced to one pint. Strain and let cool to room temperature. Wash the burn area with the tea as often as you'd like.

Aloe Vera: The juice of the aloe vera plant has been used as a burn remedy by practically every culture. Aloe vera is recommended as a remedy for burns—from sunburn to serious third-degree burns—in the literature of American Indians, New Englanders, the Amish, Indiana residents, the Romani, residents of northern Georgia, and Chinese immigrants. Aloe vera gel also acts as a disinfectant and reduces bacteria in burns.

For a small burn, break off a leaf, slice it down the middle, and rub the gel on the skin. To make a poultice of aloe, place the cut leaf on the burned area, and wrap the area with gauze. You can also apply store-bought aloe gel or juice. An alternate formula is to extend the aloe vera sap with olive oil. Here's how: Add eight ounces of extra virgin olive oil to two ounces of fresh squeezed aloe vera sap. Apply directly to the burn area.

Honey: Honey is a universal natural remedy to disinfect wounds and burns throughout the world. It is highly regarded in the literature of the Amish, Chinese immigrants, Indiana residents, and residents of the American Southwest. Honey naturally attracts water, and, when applied to a burn or wound, draws fluids out of the tissues, effectively cleaning the wound. Furthermore, most bacteria cannot live in the presence of honey. Honey is sometimes applied to gauze and used to dress severe burns in conventional medicine. In the early 1990s, physi-

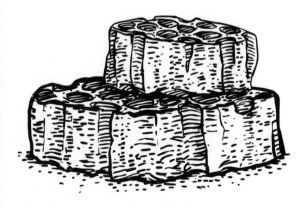

cians at a hospital in Maharashtra, India, performed clinical trials comparing honey impregnated gauze with three different conventional burn treatments, and the honey treatment was superior in each case.

In a 1991 study, the doctors compared the honey-gauze to gauze treated with silver sulfadiazine. In fifty-two patients treated with honey, ninety-one percent of wounds were sterile within seven days. In the fifty-two patients treated with silver sulfadiazine, ninety-three percent of wounds still showed signs of infection after seven days. The burns of the honey-treated patients began to heal in seven days, while for the other group, healing began on average in thirteen days. Of the wounds treated with honey, eighty-seven percent healed within fifteen days; only ten percent of the wounds healed in the control group during that time. Important: The honey also provided greater pain relief and resulted in less scarring.

You can apply honey to a piece of sterile gauze, and place directly on the burn, honey side to the skin. Change the dressing three to four times a day. Be sure to seek medical attention for serious burns.

Acne, Oily Skin, and Essential Oils

Acne may not be a hazard to your health, but it does impair your looks. The problem typically is the result of clogged skin pores. When the pores and follicles (canals that contain hair shafts) are blocked, oil cannot be secreted and builds up. Bacteria feed on the oil and multiply. People with oily skin have a greater chance of developing acne, as do teenagers and anyone experiencing hormonal fluctuations. Although not medically proven, stress may also contribute to acne breakouts.

Luckily, quite an array of essential oils is available to help you deal with acne. That's because many oils help manage the specific underlying problems that cause acne: They balance hormones, reduce stress, improve the complexion, and regulate the skin's oil production. This makes aromatherapy the ideal treatment for blemishes, pimples, and other skin eruptions. Commercial acne remedies have long recognized this.

Essential oils for acne or an oily complexion include: cedarwood, clary sage, eucalyptus, frankincense, geranium, juniper berry, lavender, lemon, lemongrass, sandalwood, and tea tree.

Toner for Oily Complexions

You will need:

- 12 drops lemongrass oil
- 6 drops juniper berry oil
- 2 drops ylang ylang oil
- 1 ounce witch hazel lotion
- 1 ounce aloe vera gel

Combine all of the ingredients in a glass bottle. Give the mixture a good shake and it's done! Apply at least once a day. If you find witch hazel too drying, vinegar is an excellent substitute. It is not as drying as the witch hazel lotion and helps to retain the skin's natural acid balance.

Zit Zap Compress

You will need:

- 4 drops cedarwood oil
- 2 drops eucalyptus oil
- 1 teaspoon Epsom salts
- ¼ cup water

Pour the boiling water over the Epsom salts. When the salts are dissolved and the water has cooled just enough to not burn the skin, add the essential oils. Soak a small absorbent cloth in the hot solution, then press the cloth against the blemishes for about one minute. Repeat several times by rewetting the cloth in the same solution.

Cuts, Scrapes, Bruises, and Essential Oils

Simple cuts and scrapes can easily be treated with antiseptic essential oils. A mist of diluted oil is an excellent way to apply them. Herbal salves containing antiseptic essential oils are also effective in treating scrapes or wounds that aren't too deep. Need to protect your cut? Many of the resins and balsams such as benzoin, frankincense, and myrrh actually form a protective barrier over the wound that acts as an antiseptic "Band-Aid."

In an emergency, don't forget that you can dab a little lavender or tea tree oil directly on a scrape as they are among the least irritating of oils.

Essential oils for cuts and scrapes include: benzoin, eucalyptus, frankincense, geranium, lavender, lemon, myrrh, rose, and tea tree.

Dermatitis, Psoriasis, Eczema, and Essential Oils

Dermatitis is an inflammation of the skin that causes itching, redness, and skin lesions. It's difficult even for dermatologists to uncover the source of this bothersome skin problem. Some obvious causes, though, are contact with an irritant such as poison oak or ivy, harsh chemicals, or anything to which one is allergic. Stress also seems to be a contributing factor in many types of dermatitis. Essential oils that counter stress, soothe inflammation and itching, soften roughness, and are both antiseptic and drying are used to treat these skin conditions.

One type of dermatitis is eczema, a word that describes a series of symptoms rather than a disease. Eczema is characterized by crusty, oozing skin that itches and may feel like it burns. Psoriasis is a dermatitis with red lesions covered by silver-like scales that flake off. This condition can be hereditary, but its cause is unknown. It has an annoying tendency to come and go for no apparent reason.

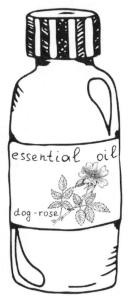

One of the best vehicles for essential oils in these cases is an herbal salve that already contains a base of skin healing herbs such as comfrey and calendula. You can use a store-bought herbal salve or one that you make yourself. Stir in 15 drops (or less) of essential oils per ounce of salve. Since salves come in a two-ounce jar, that means adding no more than 30 drops; use less if the salve already contains some essential oils. Secondary skin infections, which often occur with eczema, need to be treated with antiseptic essential oils, such as those suggested for acne.

Dermatitis Skin Care

You will need:

- 8 drops tea tree oil
- 8 drops chamomile oil
- 1 teaspoon Oregon grape tincture
- 2 ounces healing salve

With a toothpick, stir the tincture and essential oils into the salve. This will make the salve semi-liquid. You can purchase the tincture at a natural food store. Apply one to four times a day.

Dry Complexion Scrub

You will need:

- 6 drops lavender oil
- 2 drops peppermint oil
- 1 tablespoon dried elder flowers, lavender, or chamomile (optional)
- 2 tablespoons oatmeal
- 1 tablespoon cornmeal

Grind dry ingredients in a blender or electric coffee grinder. (Drugstores sell colloidal oatmeal, which needs no grinding.) Add the essential oils, and stir to distribute. Store in a closed container, and use instead of soap for cleansing your face. For clean skin, moisten 1 teaspoon with enough water to make a paste, dampen your face with a little water, then gently apply scrub. Rinse with warm water. Use this daily instead of soap.

Revitalize Your Hair

There are all types of homemade remedies you can make to improve the health of your hair. Many store-bought products can contain many harmful chemicals that do more harm to your hair than good. Below are a few useful remedies you can use to replace those damaging products you spend too much money on.

Remedies for Your Hair

❧ Eggs make a great conditioner: Beat 1 egg white until it's foamy, then stir it into 5 tablespoons of plain yogurt. Apply to your hair section by section; let sit 15 minutes. Rinse and shampoo as usual.

❧ Give your hair a conditioning treatment that will leave you feeling like you've been to an expensive salon. Mix 3 eggs, 2 tablespoons extra virgin olive oil, and 1 teaspoon distilled white vinegar. Apply to hair and cover with a plastic cap. Leave on for 30 minutes, then rinse and shampoo as usual.

❧ Use 1 tablespoon apple cider vinegar mixed with 1 gallon water as an after-shampoo rinse to minimize gray in your hair.

❧ Before shampooing, briefly soak hair in a small basin of water with 1/4 cup apple cider vinegar added. Repeat several times a week to help control dandruff and remove buildup from sprays, shampoos, and conditioners.

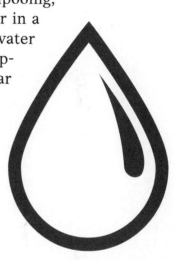

Coconut for Hair and Nails

Like healthy skin, healthy hair and nails are formed, to a great part, by a healthy diet that includes proper hydration. An unhealthy diet can lead to hair that is brittle, dull, or lifeless; a scalp that is flaky; nails that break and chip easily; and ragged cuticles. Coconut oil plays a role in radiant hair, smooth nails, and neat cuticles due to its fat content and along with coconut milk and coconut water helps hydration.

Coconut oil can be applied directly to the scalp, hair, nails, and nail beds. While excess coconut oil can be removed, the residue can remain for a healthy glow and moisturizing. Or, coconut oil can be mixed with some warm water, gently applied to the scalp, then allowed to soak into the scalp and hair before washing with shampoo and conditioner—coconut based, of course!

Plus, when coconuts are consumed they help to nourish the hair and nails from the inside out! Follow along for some of the best uses of coconut products to enrich the hair and nails.

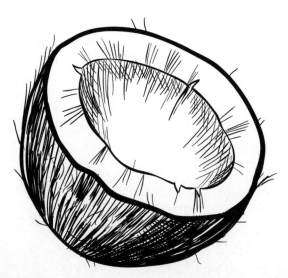

Conditions Hair

Coconut oil hydrates hair over time since it replaces the natural oils that shampoos tend to strip away. As a leave-in conditioner, coconut oil may condition the hair immediately and then benefit the hair over time. Some people think that application to wet hair is more desirable for sealing in moisture than on dry hair, but water and oil do not mix (consider vinegar and oil salad dressing), so it is best to experiment.

Dandruff Control

Dandruff along with dry scalp may be chronic problems. The daily use of coconut oil literally confronts the root of the problem. A light head massage with warm coconut oil may also be invigorating.

Reduces Split Ends

Frizzy hair is often the result of dry conditions: too many chemicals in shampoos and conditioners, coloring, perms, or general over-processing. Coconut oil helps to calm frizzy hair and restore its luster. While regular trims are best for split ends, coconut oil may tame their unruliness in the short term before a haircut.

Enhances Eyebrows and Eyelashes

Coconut oil can be used to penetrate the hair follicles in the eyebrows and eyelashes and prevent a scaly look so that they appear to be soft and shiny.

Provides Ultraviolet Protection

Sunlight helps to create a precursor of vitamin D on the skin's surface that is necessary for healthy bones and teeth, the heart, and immune function. But too much UV radiation may damage the skin and lead to some cancers. Coconut oil and its richness provide some measure of protection, but the wisest advice is to stay out of dangerous noon-day or tropical sun.

Reduces Fungal Infections

Coconut oil with its anti-microbial properties may help to prevent fungal infections of the nails (particularly toenails) and scalp. Coconut oil is even said to reduce candida, a systemic fungal infection. Make sure to check with a health care practitioner for use of specific advice.

Softens Cuticles

Coconut balm or coconut oil soothes rough and ragged cuticles before they get out of hand. When either of these nurturing coconut products is applied to the nail base, they may enhance the nails and hands.

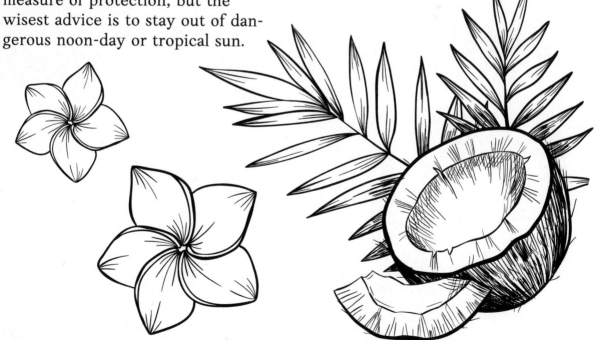

Stimulates Nail Growth

Nails need a moisturized environment in which to thrive. Coconut oil helps to prevent the nails from becoming too overly brittle and split, which may hinder their growth. Ample protein, biotin, B-complex vitamins, calcium, iron, magnesium, omega-3 fatty acids, and zinc are some of the nutrients that are needed for healthy nails.

Balances Composition of Hair and Nails

The body is a maze of natural chemicals and reactions that maintain its many functions. On low-fat diets, sometimes there is not enough fat or even protein for normal operations. Coconuts and their products may help support the body's quest for equilibrium of nutrient intake to keep it working smoothly.

Treats Hair and Scalp

Warmed coconut oil can be applied to the hair and scalp to treat dry hair before using shampoo and conditioner. The longer that it is left on the hair and scalp, the greater its moisturizing benefits. Stronger hair may be spared from dry ends that break or split up the hair and into the hair shaft.

Wards Off Infection

If used regularly, coconut oil may form a protective barrier on the skin around the nails to impede some common infections. Dry, cracked skin is more vulnerable. Make sure manicures are both safe and sanitary.

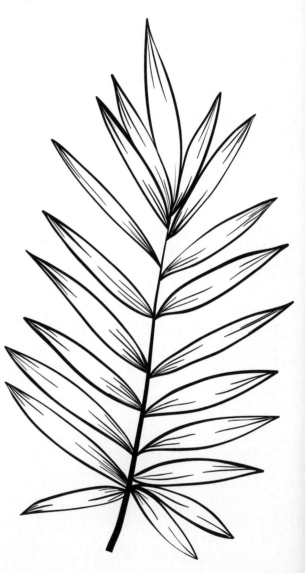

Chapter 6: More Remedies & Cures

Thus far in *Doctors' Home Remedies* we have shown you trusted cures broken down by both remedy and malady. This chapter is designed to be an antidote to the skyrocketing costs of medications and doctor visits. You'll find a wealth of additional ways to ease discomfort, treat ailments, and even prevent problems.

The painful conditions in this section are sorted alphabetically should you want to skip around. Each profile gives a short explanation of the causes and symptoms of the condition, then provides remedies categorized by type. There are dietary remedies, herbal remedies, and more.

Allergies

Approximately 40 million Americans, have seasonal allergies. But there are many other types of allergies, including animal allergy, food allergy, dust-mite allergy, and insect-sting allergy. Allergies can be called a haywire response of the immune system, which guards against intruders it considers harmful to the body, such as certain viruses and bacteria. In allergic people, however, the immune system goes a bit bonkers. It overreacts when you breathe, ingest, or touch a harmless substance. The benign culprits that trigger the overreaction, such as dust, pet dander, and pollen, are called allergens.

The body's first line of defense against invaders includes the nose, mouth, eyes, lungs, and stomach. When the immune system reacts to an allergen, it causes an inflammatory response in these battleground body parts. It releases chemicals that cause runny nose; sneezing; watery, swollen, or red eyes; nasal congestion; wheezing; shortness of breath; a tight feeling in the chest; difficulty breathing; coughing; diarrhea; nausea; headache; fatigue; and a general feeling of misery. Symptoms can occur alone or in combination and can range from mild to severe.

The tendency to become allergic is inherited, and allergies typically develop before age 30. Children with two allergic parents have a 70 percent chance of developing allergies, while children with one allergic parent have a 48 percent chance, according to the American Academy of Allergy, Asthma, and Immunology. The inherited predisposition doesn't mean you'll develop the same kind of allergy as your predecessors, however. What you become allergic to is based on the substances you are exposed to and how often you are exposed to them. Generally, the more often you encounter the allergen, the more likely it is to trigger a reaction and the greater your reaction will be.

Although allergies cannot be cured, there are plenty of ways to diminish symptoms. Allergies should be properly diagnosed by a medical doctor, particularly an allergy specialist, to avoid the inappropriate use of medications or other remedies. Many mild allergies, however, can be eased without drugs—or by a combination of self-care and pharmaceutical treatments.

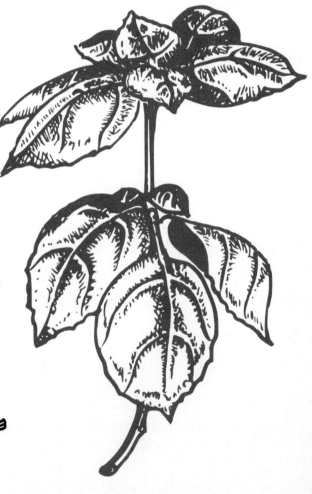

Dietary Remedies

Mint tea. Allergy sufferers throughout the centuries have turned to hot tea to relieve clogged noses and irritated mucous membranes. Mint tea is one of the best for symptom relief. It's been used by the Chinese to treat allergies since the seventh century. Mint smells delicious, and its essential oils have decongestant properties. Substances in mint also contain anti-inflammatory and mild antibacterial constituents. To make mint tea, place 1/2 ounce dried mint leaves in a 1-quart jar. Fill two-thirds of the jar with boiling water and steep for five minutes (inhale the steam). Let cool, strain, sweeten if desired, and drink.

Wasabi. If you're a hay fever sufferer and sushi lover, this remedy will please. Wasabi, that pale-green, fiery condiment served alongside California rolls, is a member of the horseradish family. Anyone who has taken too big a dollop of wasabi or plain old horseradish knows how it makes sinuses and tear ducts spring into action. That's because allyl isothiocyanate, a constituent in wasabi, promotes phlegm flow and has antiasthmatic properties. The tastiest way to get in those allyl isothiocyanates is by slathering horseradish on your sandwich or plopping wasabi onto your favorite sushi. A harder-to-swallow option is to purchase grated horseradish and take 1/4 teaspoon during an allergy attack.

Herbal Remedies

Basil. To help ease a topical allergic reaction or hives, try dousing the skin with basil tea, a traditional Chinese folk remedy. Basil contains high amounts of an anti-allergic compound called caffeic acid. Place 1 ounce dried basil leaves into 1 quart boiling water. Cover and let cool to room temperature. Use the tea as a rinse as often as needed.

Topical Remedies

Baking soda. One-half cup baking soda poured into a warm bath is an old New England folk remedy for soothing hives. Soak for 20 to 30 minutes.

Ice. Wrap a washcloth around ice cubes and apply them to your sinuses for instant relief and refreshment.

Milk. Milk does the body good, especially when it comes

to hives. Wet a cloth with cold milk and lay it on the affected area for 10 to 15 minutes.

Salt. Nasal irrigation, an effective allergy-management tool that's done right at the sink every morning, uses a mixture of salt water to rid the nasal passages of mucus, bacteria, dust, and other gunk, as well as to soothe irritated passageways. All you need is 1 to 11/2 cups lukewarm water (do not use softened water), a bulb (ear) syringe, 1/4 to 1/2 teaspoon salt, and 1/4 to 1/2 teaspoon baking soda. Mix the salt and baking soda into the water and test the temperature. To administer, suck the water into the bulb and squirt the saline solution into one nostril while holding the other closed. Lower your head over the sink and gently blow out the water. Repeat this, alternating nostrils until the water is gone. Nasal irrigation isn't a pretty sight, yet it works wonders on sore noses and rids the passages of unwanted matter.

Steam. Breathing steam refreshes and soothes sore sinuses, and it helps rid the nasal passages of mucus. It takes some time, but you will feel wonderful! Boil several cups of water and pour into a big bowl (or a plugged sink). Place your head carefully over the bowl and drape a towel over your head. Breathe gently for 5 to 10 minutes. When you're finished breathing steam, use the hot water for a second purpose. Let the water cool until warm, saturate a washcloth, and hold it on the sinuses (to the sides of your nose, below the eyes and above the eyebrows).

More Do's and Don'ts

Pass up the milk. When allergies act up, skip that extra-large, whole-milk latte since dairy products thicken mucus. Try herbal tea instead.

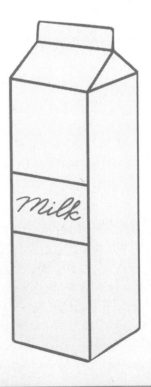

Anxiety

Anxiety is a feeling everyone experiences sooner or later. Perhaps you're sitting in the waiting room, anticipating the horse-size needle your doctor has waiting for you on the other side of the door. Or you've spent all day cooking but the look on your mother-in-law's face says your best efforts were wasted. Or you really hate your job.

These very different experiences can bring on anxiety and its typical symptoms:

- heart palpitations
- sense of impending doom
- inability to concentrate
- muscle tension
- dry mouth
- sweating
- queasy, jittery feeling in the pit of the stomach
- hyperventilation

Anxiety can be short- or long-lived, depending on its source. The more long lasting the anxiety, the more additional symptoms you will experience.

If your anxiety is a reaction to a single, isolated event (the shot the doctor is about to give you) your anxiety level will decrease and your symptoms will disappear after the event. If your anxiety is from friction between you and your mother-in-law, you're likely to experience anxiety for a period of time before and after you see her. In this case, the symptom list probably has grown to include diarrhea or constipation and irritability.

Then there's that job, a source of anxiety that never leaves you. You dread getting up in the morning because you have to go to work, dread going to bed at night because when you wake up you have to go to work, dread the weekend because when it's over you'll have to go to work. When the source of your anxiety is ever-present, you can probably add the following to the list of symptoms: chest pain, over- or under-eating, insomnia, loss of sex drive.

All three situations described above are types of everyday anxiety, or as some would put it, the cost of living. But the cost can be huge, taking its toll on you physically, mentally, and emotionally.

Although emotion is most often at the root of anxiety symptoms, they can be caused by physical problems as well. Rule out the following before assuming your symptoms are stress-related:

- Hyperthyroidism, which may produce symptoms that resemble those of anxiety
- Heart disorders, which can cause rapid heartbeat, often associated with anxiety
- Caffeine, which can produce nervous symptoms even in moderate amounts
- Premenstrual syndrome (PMS)
- Diet pills
- Anemia
- Diabetes
- Hypoglycemia

So now that you know what anxiety can do, it's time to learn what you can do to control it. Mild anxiety can be treated successfully at home with a little calming music, a little quiet time, and some soothing remedies from the kitchen.

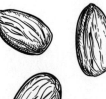

Dietary Remedies

Almonds. Soak 10 raw almonds overnight in water to soften, then peel off the skins. Put almonds in blender with 1 cup warm milk, a pinch of ginger, and a pinch of nutmeg. Drink at night to relax you before going to bed.

Orange. The aroma of an orange is known to reduce anxiety. All you have to do to get the benefits is peel an orange and inhale. You can also drop the peel into a small pan or potpourri burner. Cover with water and simmer. When heated, the orange peel will release its fragrant and calming oil.

Orange juice. For a "giddy-ap" heart rate associated with anxiety, stir 1 teaspoon honey and a pinch of nutmeg into 1 cup orange juice and drink.

Herbal Remedies

Chamomile. Sipping chamomile tea calms the nerves and aids in getting to sleep. Simply steep 1 tablespoon chamomile flowers in 1 cup water for 15 minutes, then strain and drink as needed. Breathe in its aroma, too, for a soothing effect. Use chamomile in an aroma lamp, sachet, or potpourri. However, since chamomile contains pollen, be careful if you have allergies.

Rosemary. Once used by early Californians to rid them of "evil spirits," rosemary has a calming effect on the nerves. Make a tea by adding 1 to 2 teaspoons of the dried herb to 1 cup boiling water; steep for 10 minutes, then drink. Inhaling rosemary can be relaxing, too. Burn a sprig, or use rosemary incense to ease anxiety.

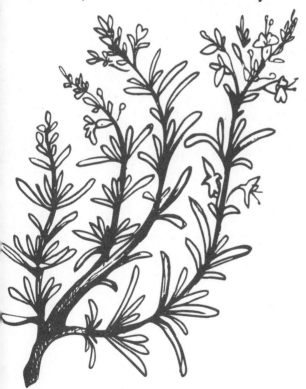

Topical Remedies

Baking soda. Add 1/3 cup baking soda and 1/3 cup ginger to a nice warm bath. Soak in the tub for 15 minutes to relieve tension and anxiety.

Ice. This is for muscle tension associated with anxiety. Wrap ice or a bag of frozen vegetables in a kitchen towel and apply it to tight muscles.

Oil. Sesame oil is great, but sunflower, coconut, or corn oil will work, too. For a wonderful, anxiety-busting massage, heat 6 ounces oil until warm, not hot. Rub over entire body, including your scalp and the bottoms of your feet. A small rolling pin feels marvelous! Use the oil as a massage before the morning bath to calm you down for the day's activities. If anxiety is keeping you awake, try using it before you go to bed, too.

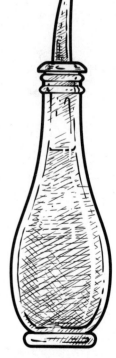

Asthma

Recent statistics about asthma don't paint a pretty picture. The National Center for Health Statistics estimates that 34 million Americans have been diagnosed with asthma in their lifetime. Almost 30 million Americans reported currently having asthma in 2007. Asthma is the number one cause of chronic illness in kids, affecting more than 6.7 million children. Despite this discouraging news, there is reason to be hopeful if you are one of the millions of asthmatics across the country. As the numbers of asthma cases continue to climb, researchers are even more determined to find asthma's causes and develop more effective treatments.

About half of all asthma attacks are caused by allergies. The most common allergens are dust mites, cockroaches, chemicals, pollen, mold, and animal dander.

In addition to allergens, asthma triggers include:

Tobacco smoke. There is a direct relationship between secondhand smoke and asthma. Secondhand smoke is a lung irritant, and it contains an abundance of harmful chemicals such as formaldehyde, arsenic, and benzene. It's especially bad for children and teenagers to be around tobacco smoke.

Exercise. Working out, especially outside in the cold, can cause exercise-induced asthma. This is not an excuse for people with asthma to shy away from exercise; they just need to consult the doctor about how to control the attacks.

Weather. Cold air can act as an asthma trigger. But other weather conditions such as rain, wind, or a sudden change in the weather can cause an attack.

Chemicals. This includes chemical fumes, such as from paint or perfume, and chemical additives, such as the sulfites that are used as preservatives in food. Any of these can trigger an asthma attack in susceptible people.

Respiratory infections. Colds, sinus infections, and even the flu can predispose one for or aggravate asthma. It's a good idea for asthmatics to get a flu shot each year.

Stomach acid. Excess stomach acid can irritate the esophagus lining and create a reaction in the lungs that may cause an attack.

Pregnancy. One-third of pregnant women with asthma get worse, but one-third of pregnant women with asthma get better, too. And one-third remain the same.

Emotional stress. Though a stressful day at work won't cause an asthma attack, it can aggravate the condition.

Drugs. Some people with asthma are sensitive to certain drugs. The most common culprits are aspirin and nonsteroidal anti-inflammatory drugs (NSAIDs).

Though there are many natural ways to help asthma sufferers breathe easier, experts recommend that combining certain natural remedies with prescription anti-inflammatories and bronchodilators are your best bet to attack your asthma. Here are some helpful remedies.

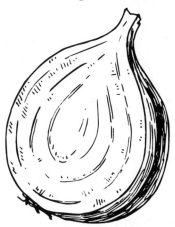

Dietary Remedies

Chili peppers. Hot foods such as chili peppers open up airways. Experts believe this happens because peppers stimulate fluids in the mouth, throat, and lungs. The increase in fluids thins out the mucus formed during an asthma attack so it can be coughed up, making breathing easier. Capsaicin, the stuff that makes hot peppers hot, acts as an anti-inflammatory when eaten and a bronchodilator when inhaled in small doses.

Coffee. The caffeine in regular coffee can help prevent and treat asthma attacks. Researchers have found that regular coffee drinkers have one-third fewer asthma symptoms than those who don't drink the hot stuff. And caffeine has bronchodilating effects. In fact, caffeine was one of the main anti-asthmatic drugs during the nineteenth century. Don't load up on java, though. Three cups per day will provide the maximum benefit.

Onions. Onions are loaded with anti-inflammatory properties. Studies have shown that these properties can reduce the constriction of the airways in an asthma attack. Use cooked onions, as raw onions are generally too irritating.

Orange juice. Vitamin C is the main antioxidant in the lining of the bronchi and bronchioles. Research discovered that people with asthma had low levels of vitamin C and that eating foods that had at least 300 mg of vitamin C per day—equivalent to about 3 glasses of orange juice—cut wheezing by 30 percent. Other foods high in vitamin C include red bell pepper, papaya, broccoli, blueberries, and strawberries.

Salmon. Fatty fish such as sardines, salmon, mackerel, and tuna contain omega-3 fatty acids. These fatty acids seem to help the lungs react better to irritants in people who have asthma and may even help prevent asthma in people who have never had an attack. Studies have found that kids who eat fish more than once a week have one-third the chance of getting asthma as children who don't eat fish. And researchers discovered that people who took fish oil supplements, equivalent to eating 8 ounces of mackerel per day, increased their body's ability to avoid a severe asthma attack by 50 percent.

Yogurt. Vitamin B12 can improve the symptoms of asthma and seems to be even more effective in asthma sufferers who are sensitive to sulfite. Studies have found that

taking 1 to 4 micrograms (mcg) works best as protection against asthma attacks. The current RDA for vitamin B12 is 2.4 mcg for adults. One cup of yogurt has 1.4 mcg of the lung-loving vitamin.

Herbal Remedies

Peppermint extract. This is a folk remedy for a homemade vaporizer. Put 1 quart nonchlorinated water in a stainless steel, glass, or enamel pan, and put it on the stove. Add 10 drops peppermint extract or peppermint oil and bring to a boil. Let it simmer for about 1 hour until all the water is gone. The volatile oil will saturate the room air.

More Do's and Don'ts

Avoid aspirin. Aspirin can trigger asthma attacks in some people. To be safe, avoid it and products that contain aspirin if you have asthma.

Take it easy on the salt. Salt tends to make the airways more sensitive to triggers.

Bad Breath

Most people are worried about having bad breath. They don't want their breath to walk into a room before they do. That's why Americans spend a billion dollars per year on mints, mouthwash, and minty-fresh toothpastes. They hope that these will prevent others from recoiling every time they speak.

More than likely, your fears of halitosis are all in your head. But if you discover your breath does have an unpleasant odor, there is usually a very treatable reason. Ninety percent of bad breath is a result of bacteria from something you ate setting up house in your mouth. Even when you brush and floss regularly, you can still miss some food particles. This can cause smelly breath.

Dietary Remedies

Fresh vegetables. Fresh vegetables, such as carrots and celery, fight plaque and keep your breath smelling nice.

Parsley. Parsley is not just for decoration. It's long been used as a breath neutralizer. Pars-ley won't get rid of bad breath, but it may help mask the garlic shrimp you had for dinner.

Sugarless gum or candy. To keep your mouth moist and increase saliva flow, the American Dental Association suggests chewing sugarless gum or sucking on sugarless candy. These are made with sorbitol, mannitol, or xylitol (sugar alcohols), which do not support oral bacterial growth.

Water. Water is essential for fresher breath. Swish water around your mouth for at least 20 seconds to loosen food particles and clean your mouth. Water may even work as well as mouthwash in removing trapped food particles and keeping your breath fresh.

Herbal Remedies

Aromatic spices. Chewing on the seeds of aromatic spices such as clove, cardamom, or fennel after meals is a common practice in South Asia and the Middle East. The seeds of these spices contain antimicrobial properties that can help halt bad breath.

Topical Remedies

Baking soda. Baking soda is a great way to clean your teeth and get fresh breath. For fresher breath, sprinkle some baking soda into your palm, dip a damp toothbrush into the baking soda, and brush.

If brushing with plain baking soda sounds icky, try adding a little artificial sugar, such as saccharine or aspartame. Or you can make your own toothpaste: Mix 3 parts baking soda with 1- part salt; add 3 teaspoons glycerin and 10 to 20 drops of your favorite flavoring (peppermint, wintergreen, anise, cinnamon); add enough water to make a paste.

To create a tooth powder, mix 3 parts baking soda with 1-part salt. Add a few drops of peppermint or wintergreen oil.

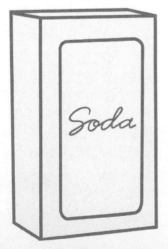

Belching

It's not a big deal, not even a medical condition most of the time. It's simply the result of swallowing air. But the air that goes down has to go somewhere, so most of the time it leaves the same way it came in, through the mouth. We all belch. Even the most prim and proper amongst us are not exempt from this oftentimes untimely eruption.

Here are some other reasons we belch:

- Belching occurs when we eat because food in the belly displaces the air that was already swallowed and is sitting in the stomach.

- Anxiety is a cause of belching, too. We get nervous, we swallow more air. The more nervous we are, the more air we swallow, and the more we belch. Anxiety belching is usually habitual and subconscious. We swallow air into the esophagus and expel it before it hits the stomach.

- An improper denture fit can cause you to swallow air.

- Drinking carbonated beverages.

- Excessive swallowing due to postnasal drip.

Medically, belching is called eructation, and the definition from *Taber's Encyclopedic Medical Dictionary* is, "Producing gas from the stomach, usually with a characteristic sound."

Dietary Remedies

Ginger. Ginger tea can help relieve the need to belch. Pour 1 cup boiling water over 1 teaspoon freshly grated gingerroot. Steep for 5 minutes, then drink.

Lemon juice. This works whether it's fresh or from the bottle. Mix 1 teaspoon lemon juice with 1/2 teaspoon baking soda in 1 cup cool water. Drink it quickly after meals.

Papaya. Most cures for belching aren't found in the fridge. But there is one surefire belch begone in the fruit drawer: papaya! It's full of an enzyme called papain that can get rid of whatever's causing that burp.

Yogurt. Eat some yogurt with live cultures (check the label) every day. It aids digestion.

Herbal Remedies

Most of the belching cures are found right here, if you know what to mix. Here are a few remedies that might just squelch that belch.

Caraway. Try some caraway seeds, straight or sprinkled on a salad. They calm the digestive tract.

Cumin. Roast equal amounts of cumin, fennel, and celery seed. Combine. After you eat, chew well about 1/2 to 1 teaspoon of the mixture, then chase it down with 1/3 cup of warm water.

Ginger. Mix 1 teaspoon fresh ginger pulp with 1 teaspoon lime juice, and take after eating.

Peppermint. Pour 1 cup boiling water over 1 teaspoon dried mint. Steep for five minutes.

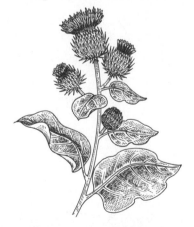

Boils

Boils have been a problem since the beginning of time. These painful bumps even got a mention in the Bible as one of the ten plagues used to convince the Egyptians to let the Israelites go. Even today, boils make people cringe. They are painful and unattractive. The good news is, though they look and feel awful, most boils are harmless. And, ironically enough, most of the treatments for boils have been around since the Egyptian doctors found themselves dealing with a boil epidemic.

Boils can appear on any part of the body that has hair follicles, but they usually occur on the face, scalp, underarm, thigh, groin, and buttocks. Boils can vary in size from small, pimple-size sores to large, painful lumps, but they are typically larger than one-half inch in diameter.

The lifetime of a boil is about two weeks. During that time the boil will grow quickly, fill with pus, and burst. After it drains, the boil needs a little tender loving care as it begins to heal.

A cluster of boils is called a carbuncle. These are most frequently found at the back of the neck or the thigh. Carbuncles are more serious than boils and are frequently accompanied by fever and fatigue. There may be whitish, bloody discharge from the carbuncle. Carbuncles require medical attention.

Dietary Remedies

Nutmeg. Nutmeg stimulates circulation in the body, which can help your body fight the bacterial infection in your boil. Stir 1/2 teaspoon ground nutmeg into 1 cup hot water and drink.

Herbal Remedies

Burdock. Burdock, which helps bring circulation to the surface of the skin, is used around the world for treating boils. Put 1 ounce dried ground burdock in 1 quart water. Bring the water to a boil and let simmer on low for 30 minutes. Drink 4 cups hot burdock tea each day until the boil comes to a head and drains. You can also apply a poultice of fresh boiled burdock leaves directly to the boil.

Chamomile. Chamomile contains antiseptic, antibacterial, and anti-inflammatory properties. To make a chamomile poultice, place 1/2 ounce chamomile flowers in a 1-pint canning jar and cover with boiling water. Cover the jar and let sit for fifteen minutes. Strain the water and apply the hot chamomile leaves directly to the boil. Cover the mash with a cloth, and be sure to keep the cloth moist with the strained liquid. Keep the leaves on for twenty minutes; repeat every two to three hours.

Chrysanthemums. Japanese researchers have discovered that chrysanthemum flowers contain properties that inhibit staphylococcus bacteria. Try using chrysanthemum tea as a poultice and drinking it as a weapon against boils.

Tea tree oil. Tea tree leaves contain a potent oil that has considerable antiseptic properties and is a very effective skin disinfectant. Research has proved that tea tree oil speeds the healing of boils, and this was attributed to its ability to inhibit staphylococcus. Tea tree oil is especially useful because it doesn't irritate the skin as it cleanses. Apply tea tree oil directly to the boil two or three times a day.

Topical Remedies

Bacon. The fat and salt content of salt pork are believed to help bring boils to a head. Roll some salt pork or bacon in salt and place the meat between two pieces of cloth. Apply the cloth to the boil. Repeat throughout the day until the boil comes to a head and drains. This can be messy.

Cornmeal. The Aztecs created a remedy for boils from dried, powdered corn flour, a remedy that is also used by the Cherokee Indians and the Appalachians. Cornmeal doesn't have medicinal properties per se, but it is absorptive, and this makes it an effective treatment for boils. Bring 1/2 cup water to a boil in a pot, and add cornmeal to make a thick paste. Apply the cornmeal mush as a poultice to the boil, and cover with a cloth. Repeat every one to two hours until the boil comes to a head and drains.

Eggs. The whites of hard-boiled eggs were used for treating boils in the nineteenth century. After boiling and peeling an egg, wet the white and apply it directly to the boil. Cover with a cloth.

Jelly jar. "Cupping" a boil, or applying suction to a boil by placing a cup or jar over the infected area, is an age-old treatment for boils. Boil a cup in a pot of water for a few minutes. Using tongs, take the cup out of the pot and let it cool down a bit before putting it over the boil (you don't want the cup to be too cool or there won't be any suction). As the cup cools over the boil, the suction brings blood and circulation to the area. Blot and wash pus away.

Milk. Heat 1 cup milk and slowly add 3 teaspoons salt (adding the salt too quickly can make the milk curdle). Simmer the milk for ten minutes. Then add flour or crumbled bread pieces to thicken the mixture. Divide the mixture into 4 poultices and apply 1 to the boil every half-hour.

Onion. The pungent onion has antiseptic chemicals and acts as an antimicrobial and irritant to draw blood and "heat" to the boil. Cut a thick slice of onion and place it over the boil. Wrap the area with a cloth. Change the poultice every three to four hours until the boil comes to a head and drains.

Bursitis

Bursitis goes by many aliases, including "Housemaid's Knee," "Clergyman's Knee," and "Baker's Cyst." Despite its nicknames, bursitis does not only affect the knee. It can hit any major joint, including the shoulder, elbow, hip, ankle, heel, or base of the big toe.

Though bursitis is associated with physical activity, you don't have to be an athlete to develop the condition. Anytime you exercise too strenuously, especially after laying off your workout for a while, you can aggravate bursitis. You can also have bursitis problems if your work or hobbies require repetitive physical movements, especially lifting things over your head. And sometimes bursitis can just flare up for no good reason.

Most cases of bursitis clear up in a couple weeks if you stop aggravating the area, but you can do a few simple things that will speed healing and make the process more comfortable. There are also some nutritional secrets that may help prevent future bursitis flare-ups.

Dietary Remedies

Orange juice. Vitamin C is a wonder nutrient. Its antioxidant properties make it an ideal addition to the diet, especially when you are recovering from an injury. Vitamin C is vital for preventing and repairing injuries and helps repair connective tissue. Not getting enough vitamin C has been found to hinder proper formation and maintenance of bursa. Men older than 19 years of age need at least 90 milligrams a day, and women older than 19 need 75 milligrams a day. However, to treat bursitis, a suggested dosage is 250 - 3,000 milligrams two times a day.

Pineapple. Pineapples contain bromelain, an enzyme that studies have shown reduces inflammation in sports injuries, such as bursitis, and reduces swelling.

Herbal Remedies

Turmeric. Studies have found that turmeric, specifically the yellow pigment in turmeric called curcumin, is a very effective anti-inflammatory. In animal studies, turmeric was as effective as cortisone, and it didn't have any side effects. Take 375 milligrams three times per day for 12 weeks. Turmeric can also increase the effects of bromelain, so they are sometimes combined or taken together. Check with your doctor first before self-treating.

Topical Remedies

Ice. Ice is a must when you're dealing with swelling. Cooling off the area slows down the blood flow and reduces inflammation. Wrap an ice pack in a thin towel and put it on the painful area for about 20 minutes.

More Do's and Don'ts

- Always warm up and stretch before doing any physical activity.
- When performing repetitive tasks, take frequent breaks.

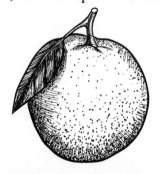

Calluses and Corns

Your poor tootsies get so little respect, but they still work hard for you. They are your foundation, and without them you wouldn't be able to chase after your toddler, walk a memo down the hall, or run in your first 5K competition. Your feet are invaluable, and they can use a little pampering. And it's better to pamper them before they start forming corns and calluses. Five percent of Americans develop corns or calluses each year, but they are avoidable.

Don't be too hard on calluses and corns. After all, their main function is protecting sensitive areas on the foot. A callus is made up of a tough protein called keratin, which is formed when dead skin cells huddle together to create a natural protection on the foot. Calluses usually form on a flat surface on the foot, such as the ball or heel. As people age, the padding on the bottom of the foot begins to thin, so a protective layer of skin naturally develops to protect the foot against too much pressure and chafing. Calluses are usually not too painful, until they get too big or too hard. Then they may start irritating the underlying skin, which can cause tenderness in the affected area.

Corns are actually a type of callus that usually forms on the toes and penetrates deeper. There are two types of corns: hard and soft. Hard corns usually form on the toe joints, such as the tops of the toes or on the outside of the pinkie toes, while soft corns form between the toes. Hard corns are described as cone-shaped because a tough core forms a tip that points inward. As with calluses, corns aren't always painful. But they are annoying and can become painful when they are irritated by chafing against each other or against the side of your shoe.

Topical Remedies

Baking soda. One of the best ways you can treat corns and calluses is with a warm-water soak. This loosens the dead skin and helps with healing. Add 3 tablespoons baking soda to a basin of warm water and soak. Or massage calluses with a paste of 3 parts baking soda to 1-part water.

Chamomile tea. Soaking your feet in diluted chamomile tea can be soothing.

Ice. Hard corns can be particularly painful. If you find yourself with a hard-core corn, apply an ice pack to the area. This will help reduce swelling and ease the pain a bit.

Cornstarch. Sprinkle cornstarch between your toes to keep the area dry. Moisture can make a corn or callus feel miserable and can promote fungal infections.

Lemon juice. Mix a paste of 1 tablespoon lemon juice and 5 or 6 crushed aspirin tablets. Apply the paste directly to your callus, and wrap your foot in a plastic bag. Keep your foot under wraps for ten minutes, allowing the acidity to soften your callus. Then give your callus a rub with a pumice stone.

Pumice stone. Pumice powder and stones are used for scouring pans and are very useful for sloughing away dead skin. After soaking your foot in warm water for about 20 minutes, use a pumice stone to rub away those corns and calluses.

Vinegar. Soak a cotton ball in vinegar and tape it to your corn or callus. Leave the vinegar-soaked cotton on overnight. In the morning, rub the area with a pumice stone.

Canker Sores

Cankers are small white sores with red edges that develop inside your mouth. They hurt like the dickens, but usually they're not serious. The most painful phase lasts about three to four days, and the sores go away in about ten days. More than 80 percent of all mouth sores are cankers, but many people confuse them with cold sores (fever blisters), which they are not. Canker sores and cold sores are two different problems altogether.

Anybody can get a canker sore, and about 20 to 60 percent of the population does at one time or another. Women are more susceptible than men, especially during their menstrual period. The first canker sore usually occurs between the ages of 10 and 40. Medical evidence also suggests that people taking certain drugs for rheumatoid arthritis may be more prone to developing cankers. And heredity is a factor, too. If both your parents were canker sore sufferers, there's a 90 percent chance you will be, too.

You can find over-the-counter antiseptic creams, lozenges, and mouthwashes at your local pharmacy to help relieve canker sore pain. There are also some home remedies that can help.

Dietary Remedies

Cranberry juice. Drink this juice between meals: It's both a pain reliever and canker healer.

Minerals and Vitamins. A mineral or vitamin deficiency is suspected of being a cause of canker sores. Make sure you get enough of minerals and vitamins in your diet, or consider taking a supplement.

Stick to cool foods. Stay away from foods that are hot (either in terms of temperature or spiciness) or that are acidic. They'll burn and sting a tender canker sore.

Herbal Remedies

Aloe. That beautiful aloe plant sitting on your windowsill has some quite potent curative powers. A little aloe juice from the juicy inner portion of the leaf rinsed over the canker several times daily could be just what you need.

Cayenne pepper. Cayenne contains capsaicin, a constituent that temporarily desensitizes the nerves that cause pain. That's why it's in a candy recipe that will relieve canker sore pain. Use the candy for relief of mouth sores from chemotherapy and radiation, too. Be careful, though, as this may be too irritating for some people.

Sage. Used most often to spice up turkey stuffing, this herb is one that can be used to calm an angry canker. Simply add 3 teaspoons sage leaves to 1 pint boiling water. Steep, covered, for 15 minutes. Rinse your mouth with the liquid several times a day. You can also rub sage leaves into a powder and apply them directly to your sore.

Topical Remedies

Baking soda. Make a baking soda and water paste and apply to the canker. Baking soda is also a component of a canker sore mouth rinse (see "Salt").

Honey. Mix 1 teaspoon honey with 1/4 teaspoon turmeric and dab it on your canker. This one may sting a bit.

Ice. This won't make the canker disappear, but it will sure make it feel better. Simply apply ice or rinse your mouth with ice water.

Salt. Combine 1 teaspoon salt, 1 teaspoon baking soda, and 2 ounces hydrogen peroxide. Mix and rinse your mouth with it four times daily. If the taste is too strong, or the tingle uncomfortable, dilute with 2 ounces water. You can also just rinse your mouth with lukewarm salt water. Or, if you're brave, just apply a little salt directly to your wound.

Tea. Moisten a regular tea bag and apply it directly to the canker. The tannic acid will help dry it out.

Colic

Bringing home a newborn baby is one of life's greatest joys. Yet it can also be one of life's greatest trials, especially if that cute little bundle of joy cries constantly. That's the number one symptom of colic: non-stop crying combined with bouts of irritability and fussiness that last a total of more than three hours per day on more than three days of the week. Colic, if it happens, typically begins at around two weeks of age and tapers off around three months. It generally is more pronounced during the evenings. Parents will be pleased to know that despite the crying, most colicky babies are healthy, well-fed infants, and the condition isn't life threatening or classified as a disease.

Unfortunately for both baby and parents, doctors don't know what causes colic, what the disorder is, or how to cure it. They don't even know if colicky babies are in pain. Fortunately for everyone involved, there are many tried-and-true ways to soothe a baby. Experiment with a few, determine what works, and stick to it.

Dietary Remedies

Basil. This aromatic herb contains large amounts of eugenol, which, among other things, has antispasmodic and sedative properties. Place 1 teaspoon dried basil leaves in a cup and fill it with boiling water. Cover and let stand for ten minutes. Strain and, while warm or at room temperature, give it to the infant in a bottle. A nursing mother may also drink the tea.

Mint. Mint has antispasmodic properties, which may help reduce intestinal spasms in colicky infants. Place 1 teaspoon dried mint in a cup and fill with boiling water. Let stand for ten minutes. Strain well and, while warm, feed to the baby in a bottle. Nursing mothers may want to have a cup of mint tea, too. A peppermint stick soaked in water may be used as an alternative, but note that many sticks contain sugar. Never use straight peppermint oil to make tea. It's too potent for a baby.

Soy products. That carton of cow's milk looks innocent enough, but it can be the problem source for five to ten percent of colicky babies. Many studies have shown an improvement in colic after dairy products have been eliminated from babies' diets. The culprit seems to be the proteins in cow's milk. (Don't think milk is the only villain. This protein lurks in many infant formulas containing dairy and is also found in the milk of breast-feeding mothers who consume dairy products.) Try eliminating dairy products for two weeks and switch to soy products, both for baby and for you if you're breast-feeding. If you don't notice any improvement, milk probably isn't the culprit.

Herbal Remedies

Chamomile tea. Chamomile combines antispasmodic and sedative properties and may relieve intestinal cramping and induce relaxation at the same time. In fact, chamomile contains 19 different antispasmodic constituents, as well as 5 sedative ones. To make a cup of tea: Place 1 teaspoon chamomile flowers in a cup and fill with boiling water. Cover and let stand for ten minutes. Strain and, while warm or at room temperature, give to the infant in a bottle. A nursing mother may also drink the tea, unless she is allergic to pollens. Prepackaged chamomile tea bags may be used instead of flowers.

Topical Remedies

Warm water. Put warm (not hot) water in a hot water bottle and place it against your baby's stomach. This can be soothing.

Constipation

Constipation occurs for many different reasons. Stress, lack of exercise, certain medications, artificial sweeteners, and a diet that's lacking fiber or fluids can each be the culprit. Certain medical conditions such as an underactive thyroid, irritable bowel syndrome, diabetes, and cancer also can cause constipation. Even age is a factor. The older we get, the more prone we are to the problem.

Some people mistakenly believe they must have a certain number of bowel movements per day or per week or else they are constipated. That couldn't be further from the truth, although it's a common misconception. What constitutes "normal" is individual and can vary from three bowel movements a day to three a week. You'll know if you're constipated because you'll be straining a lot in the bathroom, you'll produce unusually hard stools, and you'll feel gassy and bloated.

It's not a good idea to use laxatives as the first line of attack when you're constipated. They can become habit-forming to the point that they damage your colon. Some laxatives inhibit the effectiveness of medications you're already taking, and there are laxatives that cause inflammation to the lining of the intestine.

Conventional thinking on laxatives is that if you must take one, find one that's psyllium- or fiber-based. Psyllium is a natural fiber that's much gentler on the system than ingredients in many of the other products available today. Or, simply look in the kitchen for relief.

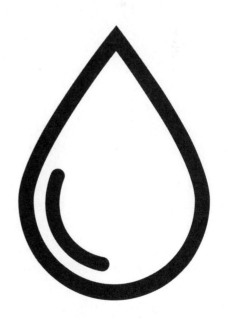

Dietary Remedies

Apples. Eat an hour after a meal to prevent constipation.

Apple juice, apple cider. These are natural laxatives for many people. Drink up and enjoy!

Bananas. These may relieve constipation. Try eating two ripe bananas between meals. Avoid green bananas because they're constipating.

Barley. It can relieve constipation as well as keep you regular, and it has cholesterol-lowering properties, too. What more could you ask of a simple grain? Buy some barley flour, flakes, and grits. Add some barley grain to vegetable soup or stew.

Blackstrap molasses. Take 2 tablespoons before going to bed. It has a pretty strong taste, so you may want to add it to milk, fruit juice, or for an extra-powerful laxative punch, prune juice.

Fiber. Sometimes all you need to ensure regularity is some extra fiber in your diet. Fiber is the indigestible part of plant foods, and it adds mass to the stool and stimulates the colon to push things along. It's found naturally in fruits, vegetables, grains, and beans. The current recommendations for daily dietary fiber are 20 to 35 grams a day, but most people eat only 10 to 15 grams. Fiber supplements may be helpful, but you're better off getting your fiber from foods, which supply an assortment of other essential nutrients as well. To avoid getting gassy, increase the fiber in your diet gradually, and be sure to drink plenty of water so the fiber can move smoothly through your digestive system.

Garlic. In the raw, it has a laxative effect for many. Eat it mixed with onion, raw or cooked, and with milk or yogurt for best results.

Honey. This is a very mild laxative. Try taking 1 tablespoon three times per day, either by itself or mixed into warm water. If it doesn't work on its own, you may have to pep it up by mixing it half and half with blackstrap molasses.

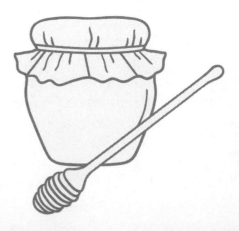

Oil. Safflower, soybean, or other vegetable oil can be just the cure you need, as they have a lubricating action in the intestines. Take 2 to 3 tablespoons a day until the problem is gone. If you don't like taking it straight, mix the oil with herbs and lemon juice or vinegar to use as salad dressing. The combination of the oil and the fiber from the salad ought to fix you right up.

Raisins. Eat a handful daily, an hour after a meal.

Rhubarb. This is a natural laxative. Cook it and eat it sweetened with honey or bake it in a pie. Or, create a drink with cooked, pureed rhubarb, apple juice, and honey.

Walnuts. Fresh from the shell, they may be just the laxative you need.

Herbal Remedies

Flaxseeds. These provide natural bulk and will relieve constipation. Wash 2 teaspoons seeds in cold water. Add to 1 cup boiling water. Let steep for ten minutes, then drink. Do not strain out the seeds.

Senna. This will work, but children under 12 and women who are pregnant should not use it. Here's the recipe: Place 1/4 to 1/2 teaspoon crushed senna leaves or powder in 1 cup boiling water. Let it steep for ten minutes. Use once a day for no more than ten days. Warning! Use only a small amount of senna. It's very strong, and one full teaspoonful can cause abdominal cramping.

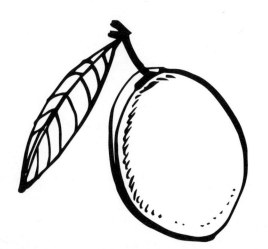

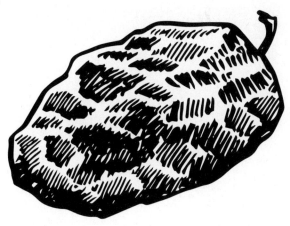

Cough

Annoying, loud, and disruptive, a persistent cough can put a damper on your daily routine. Coughs can be defined by how long they last. A brief cough is caused by such factors as cold air, irritating fumes, breathing dust, or drawing food into the airways. A persistent cough, however, typically results from mucus and other secretions brought on by respiratory disorders such as the cold, the flu, pneumonia, or tuberculosis.

Regardless of time and moisture content, a cough is produced when viruses, bacteria, dust, pollen, or other foreign substances irritate respiratory passages in the throat and lungs. The cough reflex is the body's effort to rid the passageways of such intruders, and it spares no power in the expulsion. A cough reflex can expel a foreign substance at velocities as high as 100 miles per hour.

Determine what kind of cough you have and search out cures specific to that type. Some remedies aim to moisten dry throats, while others are expectorants, helping you cough up and get rid of mucus and irritants. Most of these cures aim to battle both coughs unless otherwise noted.

Dietary Remedies

Chicken soup. Take some advice from your grandma: Sip a bowl of chicken soup. It doesn't matter if it's homemade or canned. Chicken soup is calming for coughs associated with colds. Although scientists can't put a finger on why this comfort food benefits the cold sufferer, they do believe chicken soup contains anti-inflammatory properties that help relieve a cold's miserable side effects, one being the cough. Plus, chicken soup contains cysteine, which thins phlegm. The broth, chock-full of electrolytes, keeps you hydrated, and the steam helps soothe irritated mucous membranes and air passageways. Last, but not least, it tastes yummy.

Honey. Honey has long been used in traditional Chinese medicine for coughs because it's a natural expectorant, promoting the flow of mucus. This is the simple recipe: Mix 1 tablespoon honey into 1 cup hot water and enjoy. Now how sweet is that? Squeeze some lemon juice in if you want a little tartness.

Licorice. If you love licorice, you're in for a treat with this remedy. Many folk remedies use licorice root to treat coughs and bronchial problems. It serves not only as a flavoring agent but also as a demulcent (a substance that soothes inflamed or irritated throats) and an expectorant. Real licorice or candy that's made with real licorice (look for licorice mass on the label) works best. Reach into your candy jar and slice up 1 ounce licorice sticks. Add 1 quart boiling water and steep for 24 hours. Drink throughout the day, adding a teaspoon of honey for sweetness.

Herbal Remedies

Garlic. Eating garlic won't have you winning any kissing contests, but who wants to kiss you when you sound like a seal? Garlic is full of antibiotic and antiviral properties, plus garlic is also an expectorant, so it helps you cough up stubborn bacteria and/or mucus that are languishing in your lungs.

Ginger. Ginger, which has antiviral properties, shares the limelight with licorice in this cough remedy. To make ginger-licorice (anise) tea, combine 2 teaspoons freshly chopped ginger root, 2 teaspoons aniseed, and if available, 1 teaspoon dried licorice root in 2 cups boiling water. Cover and steep for ten minutes. Strain and sweeten with

1 or 2 teaspoons honey. Drink 1/2 cup every one to two hours, but no more than 3 cups per day.

Mustard seed. An irritating but useful spice for wet coughs, mustard seed has sulfur-containing compounds that stimulate the flow of mucus. To get the full effect of the expectorant compounds, the mustard seeds must be broken and allowed to sit in water for 15 minutes. Crush 1 teaspoon mustard seeds or grind them in a coffee grinder. Place the seeds in a cup of warm water. Steep for 15 minutes. This concoction might be a little hard to swallow, so take it in 1/4-cup doses throughout the day.

Pepper. Pepper is an irritant (try sniffling some), but this characteristic is a plus for those suffering from coughs accompanied by thick mucus. The irritating property of pepper stimulates circulation and the flow of mucus in the airways and sinuses. Place 1 teaspoon black pepper into a cup and sweeten things up with the addition of 1 tablespoon honey. Fill with boiling water, steep for 10 to 15 minutes, stir, and sip.

Thyme. Store-bought cough syrups are often so medicinal tasting that it's hard to get them down without gagging. Here's a sweet, herbal version, made of thyme, peppermint, mullein, licorice, and honey, that's guaranteed to go down the hatch easily. Thyme and peppermint help clear congested air passages and have antimicrobial and antispasmodic properties to relieve the hacking. Mullein and licorice soothe irritated membranes and help reduce inflammation.

To make the syrup, combine 2 teaspoons each dried thyme, peppermint, mullein, and licorice root into 1 cup boiling water. Cover and steep for half an hour. Strain and add 1/2 cup honey. If the honey doesn't dissolve, heat the tea gently and stir. Store in the refrigerator in a covered container for as long as three months. Take 1 teaspoon as needed.

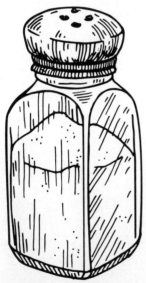

Topical Remedies

Salt. A saltwater gargle is a simple solution to a cough, although you have to remain devoted to gargling to get results. Mix 1/4 teaspoon salt into 4 ounces warm water. Mix and gargle. Repeat this every one to two hours each day for best results. The salt, combined with soothing warm water, acts as an astringent to help ease irritated and inflamed throat tissues and loosen mucus.

Steam. One of the kitchen's best remedies for a cough is also one of the easiest. Inhaling steam helps flush out mucus, and it moisturizes dry, irritated air passageways. Fill a cooking pot one-quarter full with water. Boil, turn off the heat, and if available, add a couple drops essential oil of eucalyptus. Carefully remove the pot from the stove, and place it on a protected counter or table. Drape a towel over your head, lean over the pot, and breathe gently for 10 to 15 minutes. Don't stick your face too far into the pot or you'll get a poached nose.

Dehydration

Every cell in your body needs water in order to function properly. In fact, an adult's body weight is 60 percent water while an infant's is as much as 80 percent water. Other than oxygen, there's nothing that your body needs more than water. Water is so important because it has many critical functions in the body.

Each and every time you exhale, water escapes your body, as much as 2 cups per day. It evaporates invisibly from your skin, another 2 cups a day. And you urinate approximately 2 1/2 pints every 24 hours. Add it up, and you could be losing up to 10 cups of water every day, and that's before you break a sweat.

Because water has so many life-sustaining functions, dehydration isn't just a matter of being a little thirsty. The effects depend on the degree of dehydration, but a water shortage causes your kidneys to conserve water, which in turn can affect other body systems. You'll urinate less and you can become constipated.

How much water do you need each day? Under normal conditions, the standard of 64 ounces a day is sufficient. That amount includes water from sources other than the tap. If you're an athlete or someone who spends a lot of time out in the sun sweating, you'll probably need more. A good way to tell if you're adequately hydrated is by observing the color of your urine. If it's dark yellow or amber, that's a sign that it's concentrated, meaning there's not enough water in the wastes that are being eliminated. If it's light, the color of lemon juice, that's normal.

The simple cure for dehydration comes from the tap. Turn it on and drink. But there are other helpers that will keep you hydrated, too.

Dietary Remedies

Bananas. They have great water content and are especially good for restoring potassium that has vanished with dehydration.

Bland foods. If you're experiencing dehydration, stick to foods that are easily digested for the next 24 hours because stomach cramps are a symptom and can recur. Try saltines, rice, bananas, potatoes, and flavored gelatins. Gelatins are especially good since they are primarily made of water.

Decaffeinated tea. Just another tasty way to get fluids in your body. Don't drink caffeinated tea, however, as caffeine is a mild diuretic.

Fruit juice. It's liquid and has essential vitamins and minerals that need to be replenished.

Ice. Suck on it, or rub it on your body when you're overheated. This will help cool you down and prevent excess evaporation, which may lead to dehydration.

Lime juice. Add 1 teaspoon lime juice, a pinch of salt, and 1 teaspoon sugar to a pint of water. Sip the beverage throughout the day to cure mild dehydration.

Popsicle. A great way to restore water to your body. It's an easy way to get fluids into kids, too.

Raisins. They're packed with potassium, a body salt lost during dehydration.

Salt. If you're experiencing symptoms of mild dehydration or heat injury, or you're just plain sweating a lot, make sure you replace your salt. Don't just chug salt straight from the box, however. Try eating pretzels, salted crackers, or salty nuts.

Sports drinks. Not only will they add water back into your system, they'll restore potassium and other essential electrolytes (a salt substance, such as potassium, sodium, and chlorine found in blood, tissue fluids, and cells that carry electrical impulses). For children, these adult drinks may be too harsh, so talk to your pharmacist about pediatric rehydration drinks now on the market.

Watery fruits. Bananas are the number one fruit for rehydration, but watery fruits are a delicious and nutritious way to restore fluids. Try cantaloupe, watermelon, and strawberries. Watery vegetables such as cucumbers are good, too.

Yogurt. Or cottage cheese. These have both sodium and potassium for replacing electrolytes.

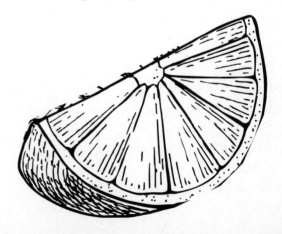

Topical Remedies

Salt. To slough off the dry, flaky skin that comes from dehydration, try this: After you bathe and while your skin is still wet, sprinkle salt onto your hands and rub it all over your skin. This salt massage will remove dry skin and make your skin smoother to the touch. It will also invigorate your skin and get your circulation moving.

Also, if your skin is itchy as a result of dehydration, soaking in a tub of salt water can be a great itchy skin reliever. Just add 1 cup table salt or sea salt to bathwater. This solution will also soften skin and relax you.

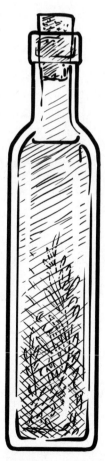

Vinegar. Since achy muscles are a side effect of dehydration, this can bring relief. Add 8 ounces apple cider vinegar to a bathtub of warm water. Soak in tub for at least 15 minutes.

Diabetes

Diabetes is a disease that reduces, or stops, the body's ability to produce or respond to insulin, a hormone produced in the pancreas. Insulin's role is to open the door for glucose, a form of sugar, to enter the body's cells so that it can be used for energy. When the body has a problem metabolizing glucose, it builds up in the blood, and the body's cells starve.

There is no cure for diabetes, but it can be controlled. And control is essential because diabetes can lead to heart disease, stroke, kidney disease and failure, blindness, and amputation if not treated. This profile will not address diabetic medical treatment, including prescribed diabetic diets. Those specifics must be left up to your physician and dietitian. Before you try any alternative practice, consult your physician. Nothing contained in this profile is intended to stop or replace your prescribed diabetic care!

Dietary Remedies

Asparagus. This vegetable is a mild diuretic that's said to be beneficial in the control of diabetes. Eat it steamed and drizzled with olive oil and lemon juice.

Lemon. A tasty substitute for salt. It's great squeezed into a diet cola, too. It cuts the aftertaste.

Olive oil. Studies indicate this may reduce blood sugar levels. Use it in salad dressing or wherever cooking oils are indicated. For an inexpensive and easy no-stick olive oil spray-on coating, buy an oil mister in any department store kitchen supply area and use it to spray your pans before cooking.

Oolong tea. Drinking oolong tea combined with taking hypoglycemic drugs may be an effective treatment for type 2 diabetes. Participants in a 2003 study of Taiwanese adults with diabetes were given either six cups of oolong tea or water per day, along with blood glucose-lowering medications. After one month, the glucose levels of those given the oolong tea were significantly reduced compared to those given water alone.

Peanut butter. After you've experienced an episode of low blood sugar and corrected it, follow up with a protein and carbohydrate snack. Peanut butter on a couple of crackers supplies both, and it's easy to fix when you may still feel a little jittery. Just avoid brands that contain added sugar, glucose, or jelly.

Salt. Set the salt shaker aside, put it back in the cupboard, hide it. High blood pressure is a side effect of diabetes, and that means salt's a no-no. If it's out of sight, or inconvenient to get, you might just skip it. Instead, reach for an herb or spice blend that's sodium free. Make one yourself with your favorite spices or buy one at the store.

Sugar. Yes, even people with diabetes need it occasionally when their blood sugar goes too low. A spoonful of straight sugar will work, as will a piece of hard candy. Just be sure it's not sugarless.

Vinegar. Muscle cramps, especially in the legs, can affect people with diabetes. For relief from the ache, add 8 ounces apple cider vinegar to a bathtub of warm water. Soak for at least 15 minutes.

Herbal Remedies

Parsley. Steep into a tea and drink. This may act as a diuretic as well as lower blood sugar.

Watercress. This is said to strengthen the natural defense systems of people who have diabetes. It's also a mild diuretic. Wash the leaves thoroughly, and add them to a salad. Or smear a little cream cheese on a slice of bread, then top with watercress for a delicious open-faced sandwich.

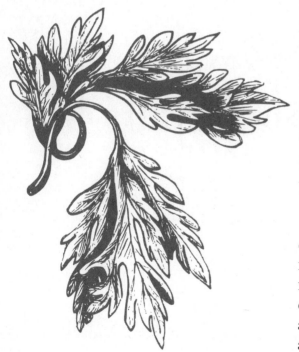

Diarrhea

Diarrhea is probably one of the most unpleasant problems that plagues us, and it's a common malady. Americans usually suffer from diarrhea a couple times a year. For most adults, diarrhea isn't serious. And it does give you a chance to ponder some redecorating ideas for the bathroom.

On a typical day, you eat a meal and the food makes its way through the digestive system without any problems. By the time it reaches the intestines, your food is mostly fluid with bits of solid material. The intestines reabsorb most of the fluid, and the solid stuff is excreted in the usual fashion. But when you've got diarrhea, something blocks the intestine's ability to absorb fluid. You've got loads of watery fluids mixed in with your stool, and you get that "gotta go" feeling.

There are essentially two types of diarrhea: acute and chronic. Thankfully, the vast majority of diarrhea is acute, or short term. This type of diarrhea keeps you on the toilet for a couple of days but doesn't stick around long. Acute diarrhea is also known as non-inflammatory diarrhea. Its symptoms are what most people associate with the condition: watery, frequent stools accompanied by stomach cramps, gas, and nausea.

Acute diarrhea usually has a bacterial or viral culprit. Gastroenteritis, mistakenly called the "stomach flu," is one of the most common infections that cause diarrhea. Gastroenteritis can be caused by many different viruses. Eating or drinking foods contaminated with bacteria can also cause diarrhea. Other causes of acute diarrhea are lactose intolerance, sweeteners such as sorbitol, over-the-counter antacids that contain magnesium, too much vitamin C, and some antibiotics.

If you have chronic, or long-term, diarrhea that comes on suddenly and stays for weeks, you may have a more serious condition such as irritable bowel syndrome or a severe food allergy.

With any kind of diarrhea, you lose a lot of fluids. One of the quickest ways you can end up going from the bathroom to the emergency room is to take a pass on liquids while you're sick. Fluids not only keep things running smoothly in your body, they also keep electrolyte levels balanced. Your body needs electrolytes such as sodium, potassium, and chloride salts for proper

organ function. An electrolyte imbalance can cause your heart to beat irregularly, causing life-threatening problems. Though drinking or eating anything while you're running back and forth to the bathroom might sound grotesque, it will help make you more comfortable and get you back on your feet more quickly.

Though experts don't see eye to eye on what fluids are best during a bout with diarrhea, they do agree that getting two to three quarts of fluid per day is a good idea. When you drink, it's easier on the tummy if you sip instead of gulp and if you drink cool, not cold or hot, fluids. Here are some tried-and-true fluids that should get you through the rough days.

- Decaffeinated tea with a little sugar
- Sports drinks
- Commercially available electrolyte replacement drinks for children
- Bouillon
- Chicken broth
- Orange juice

Though it may not sound logical to put diarrhea and food in the same sentence, if you don't put something in your body while you're enduring tummy troubles, you might end up getting sicker. There are loads of good things from the kitchen that will ease your grumbling stomach, and there are a few things that will prevent those diarrhea-causing agents from coming back for a return engagement.

Dietary Remedies

Banana. Long known as a soother for tummy trouble, this potassium-rich fruit can restore nutrients and is easy to digest.

Blueberries. Blueberry root is a long-time folk remedy for diarrhea. In Sweden, doctors prescribe a soup made with dried blueberries for tummy problems. Blueberries are rich in anthocyanosides, which have antioxidant and antibacterial properties, as well as tannins, which combat diarrhea.

Cooked cereals. Starchy foods, such as precooked rice or tapioca cereals, can help ease your tummy. Prepare the cereal according to the directions on the box, making it as thick as you can stomach it. Just avoid adding too much sugar or salt, as these can aggravate diarrhea. It's

probably a good idea to avoid oatmeal since it's high in fiber and your intestines can't tolerate the added bulk during a bout with diarrhea.

Orange peel. Orange peel tea is a folk remedy that is believed to aid in digestion. Place a chopped orange peel (preferably from an organic orange, as peels otherwise may contain pesticides and dyes) into a pot and cover with 1 pint boiling water. Let it stand until the water is cooled. You can sweeten it with sugar or honey.

Potatoes. This is another starchy food that can help restore nutrients and comfort your stomach. But eating french fries won't help. Fried foods tend to aggravate an aching tummy. Other root vegetables such as carrots (cooked, of course) are also easy on an upset stomach, and they are loaded with nutrients.

Rice. Cooked white rice is another starchy food that can be handled by someone recovering from diarrhea.

Yogurt. Look for yogurt with live cultures. These "cultures" are friendly bacteria that can go in and line your intestines, providing you protection from the bad guys. If you've already got diarrhea, yogurt can help produce lactic acid in your intestines, which can kill off the nasty bacteria and get you feeling better, faster.

Herbal Remedies

Chamomile tea. Chamomile is good for treating intestinal inflammation, and it has antispasmodic properties as well. You can brew yourself a cup of chamomile tea from packaged tea bags, or you can buy chamomile flowers and steep 1 teaspoon of them and 1 teaspoon of peppermint leaves in a cup of boiling water for fifteen minutes. Drink 3 cups a day.

Fenugreek seeds. Science has given the nod to this folk remedy, but only for adults. Mix 1/2 teaspoon fenugreek seeds with water and drink up.

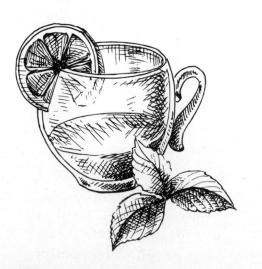

More Do's and Don'ts

❧ Don't take antidiarrheal medications at the onset of your illness. Let your body rid itself of whatever's causing the problem first.

❧ Wash your hands thoroughly before preparing food. You don't want to pass your illness to everyone in the household.

Dry Mouth

Dry mouth, also known as xerostomia, is a condition in which saliva production shuts down. When working at full capacity, saliva has many duties. This versatile fluid helps us talk, chew, and spit. It acts as a natural cavity fighter by washing away food particles and plaque, and it helps to digest food, works to buffer acids, and remineralizes those pearly whites. Saliva is vital in maintaining a healthy mouth, so when production decreases or stops, there is more than a dry mouth to pout about. Teeth and gums become more prone to decay and infection, and your taste buds might suffer, too.

Dehydration is an obvious cause of dry mouth. However, dehydration doesn't always arise from obvious reasons. You can become dehydrated through fever, extensive exercise, vomiting, diarrhea, burns, and blood loss. Other causes of xerostomia are radiation therapy, menopause, surgical removal of the salivary glands, and cigarette smoking.

Dietary Remedies

Celery sticks. If you need an excuse to snack, here it is! Munching on such waterlogged snacks as celery sticks helps stimulate the saliva glands and adds moisture to your mouth. Should your sweet tooth strike, suck on sugarless candies. Definitely stay away from sugar-filled treats since they promote decay in an already vulnerable mouth.

Liquids. If the salivary glands are down for the count, you'll need all the reinforcements you can muster to help get food down. Try to complement each dish with sauce, gravy, broth, butter, or yogurt. Food will be easier to swallow. Another option is to stick to soft, liquid-based foods, such as stews, soups, and noodle dishes.

Parsley. A dry mouth is not only uncomfortable, but it often brings out bad breath. This double whammy can ruin just about any social situation. Luckily, battling bad breath is easy. See that parsley on your plate? The restaurant may put it there for decoration, but it can serve a more useful purpose. This herb is a natural breath sweetener, and it provides ample amounts of vitamins A and C, calcium, and iron. So, chew on some.

Herbal Remedies

Aniseed. Munching on aniseed can help combat the bad breath that accompanies dry mouth. In fact, many Indian restaurants have a bowl of anise and fennel available to remove pungent food odors from your breath. Mix a few teaspoons of these seeds, place in a covered bowl, and keep on the table.

Cayenne pepper. A dry mouth often inhibits taste buds from distinguishing between sour, sweet, salty, and bitter flavors. A mouth-watering method to stimulate saliva production and bolster those buds is to sprinkle red pepper (cayenne) on your food or mix it into your favorite juice (tomato juice seems most compatible). Better yet, prepare an entire meal around red pepper, which acts as nature's wake-up call, stimulating salivary glands, sweat glands, and tear ducts.

Fennel. Munching on fennel seeds mixed with aniseed can help combat bad breath that accompanies dry mouth. In addition, fennel seed can be combined with other herbs to make a mouthwash.

Rosemary. Store-bought mouthwash overflows with germ-killing alcohol, which is also a drying agent. Read labels and don't purchase any that contain alcohol. Better yet, reach into your spice rack and pull out rosemary, mint, and aniseed to make a refreshing herbal mouthwash. The rosemary helps fight germs, while the mint and aniseed freshen breath. Combine 1 teaspoon dried rosemary, 1 teaspoon dried mint, and 1 teaspoon aniseed with 2 1/2 cups boiling water. Cover and steep for 15 to 20 minutes. Strain and refrigerate. Use as a gargle.

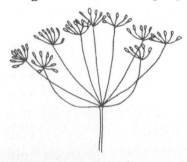

Eye Puffiness

Do you wake up looking as if you cried all night? Are your eyes so swollen when you come home from work that your significant other thinks you spent the day at the pub instead? Swollen, red eyes can make life miserable, not to mention cause others to misinterpret your lifestyle. Using a little insight, however, can help determine the cause of marshmallow eyes. A diet dominated by salty foods and allergies or chronic sinusitis are two common reasons for eye puffiness. Oftentimes, what you can't see can bother you. Irritants and chemicals found in make-up, perfumes, and detergents can have inflammatory effects on eyes. And eyes definitely don't take kindly to today's computer-focused workplace; they rebel with redness.

But look at it this way: Puffy eyes are only a temporary problem for most people. Many cases can be cured by simple home remedies and/or by eliminating substances that may cause swelling.

Dietary Remedies

Drinking water. Water is the saving grace when it comes to reducing eye puffiness. Be sure you drink at least eight, 8-ounce glasses of water each day, and don't substitute sodas, coffees, or sugary drinks. When the body is dehydrated, it acts much like a camel, storing water for the long haul across the desert. Instead of a camel's hump, you'll develop water reserves around the eyeballs. By keeping yourself adequately hydrated, the body isn't put into survival mode and won't puff up in all the wrong places.

Topical Remedies

Cold water. Eyes seem to puff up on workday mornings when you have 30 minutes to get ready. There's no time to luxuriate with tea bags and cucumber slices—but don't despair. Cold water will work in a pinch. Rise, shine, and rinse your face with several splashes of cold water. This may be a rude awakening, but the coldness will constrict blood vessels and reduce swelling. Plus, it only takes ten seconds. Repeat throughout the day if possible. Just remember to wear waterproof eye makeup.

Cucumbers. From the vegetable bin comes the well-known cucumber remedy. Cucumbers aren't only deliciously cool and soothing to the touch, but their astringent properties cause blood vessels to constrict. Lean your head back, rest a slice on each closed eye, and relax for five to ten minutes while the cukes cure your puffiness.

Egg whites. Call this kitchen cure a soufflé for the face. Whip up 1 or 2 egg whites until stiff and apply with a brush or soft cloth underneath your eyes. The skin will feel tighter and look less like puff pastry.

Potato. The common potato also pampers puffy eyes. Tubers are tried and true in European folk medicine as a means to soothe painful joints, headaches, and other inflammatory conditions. Potato starch acts as an anti-inflammatory agent to ease irritated eyes. Start by pretending you're making hash browns. Peel one potato, wash and dry it. Grate the potato as fine as possible, then instead of frying it up with butter, place the pulp in a clean cloth and fold to make a poultice. Place the poultice on your eyelids for 15 minutes.

Salt. Jumbo fries, pepperoni pizza, and other salt-infested foods can cause puffy eyes. However, salt by itself does the eyes good. Get rid of the puffy eye façade by mixing 1/2 teaspoon salt into 1 quart warm water. Dip cotton balls or facial pads into the solution, then lie down and apply pads to the eyelids. Rest in this position for at least ten minutes while keeping the pads in place. You'll arise with deflated eyes.

Spoons. Teaspoon-size spoons are just the right utensils for temporarily helping your eyes reduce to normal proportions. Place 4 (or 6) spoons in the refrigerator. When you need to deflate those eyeballs, lie down, close your eyes, and place one spoon (curved side down) on each eye. As the spoon warms, replace it with a cold one from the fridge.

Tea. Green tea or black? Both work well to soothe puffy, irritated eyes. The difference? Not much. Caffeinated teas help constrict blood vessels and reduce swelling, while herbal teas (especially chamomile) contain anti-irritants that soothe redness and inflammation. Steep 2 bags of your choice of tea in hot water for three to five minutes. Let cool until the bags are comfortably warm to the touch. Lie down, close your eyes, and place a tea bag over each eye; then cover with a soft cloth. During hot months, put the cooked tea bags in the refrigerator and apply to eyes when needed for a refreshing, eye-opening experience.

Flatulence

Who is the most glamorous person you know? Well, that person's not exempt from this particular problem. No one is. And it happens at the most awkward times, doesn't it? You feel that rumble way down deep in your belly, and it's traveling even lower. In the middle of very polite company it gurgles inside, and you glance at the person next to you so no one will know that the undertone of the impending blast belongs to you.

Well, gas happens. Called flatus, or flatulence when it finally does escape, it's normal. Its beginnings are in the foods we eat. We eat, therefore we pass gas. Why? Our stomach acids are breaking down last night's pasta primavera into elements that will either be absorbed into the body or eliminated. And that breakdown causes...You guessed it: Gas!

Bodily gas originates in the stomach and travels down to the intestines. Its construction is pretty simple: carbon dioxide, hydrogen, nitrogen, and methane. Well, those gases make up about 99 percent of the gas we pass. The other 1 percent is divided among as many as 250 different gases, all of which occur naturally when carbohydrates are broken down. If you swallow air, you add oxygen to the mix.

Not all flatulence has an unpleasant odor, but some eye-watering "squeakers" can be enough to make you haul out the old gas mask. As bacteria in the gut munches on certain foods, it produces distinctly stinky gases. Humans pass gas, on average, 14 to 23 times each day.

Gas is a side effect or symptom, not an illness in itself. And it's a symptom that can be treated several different ways with things you find in the kitchen.

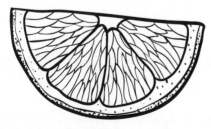

Dietary Remedies

Caraway crackers. Caraway seeds and their oils are carminatives (they get rid of gas), but who wants to eat just the seeds? Caraway seed crackers and breads with caraway seeds are a tasty way to make your system gas-unfriendly.

Citrus fruits. Vitamin C in tablet form may cause gas, especially amounts in excess of 500 milligrams. So, reduce the dosage and replace the C with high-in-C fruits. Also try potatoes and sweet peppers, which are high in vitamin C.

Minimize milk consumption. Some people don't have enough of the enzyme lactase in their gut to digest lactose, the sugar in milk. If you are lactose intolerant, replace the milk in your diet with calcium-fortified orange juice or with calcium-fortified soy milk. Or try lactose-reduced milk, which is available at your grocer.

Pumpkin. It soothes the tummy, and best of all, it cuts down on flatulence. Try some baked, steamed, or broiled. Or make yourself a simple pumpkin soup.

Well-cooked beans. Beans that are undercooked are more likely to cause gas than beans that are well-cooked. To ensure that your beans are cooked thoroughly, pull out the pressure cooker and follow the manufacturer's advice for cooking beans. Or, cook them up to pressure for 30 minutes at 15 pounds per square inch on the gauge.

Yogurt with acidophilus. It alleviates digestive woes, including gas. But the yogurt must have live acidophilus, a bacteria that helps with digestion.

Herbal Remedies

Cardamom seeds. These speed digestion. Add them to sautéed vegetables or to rice or lentils before cooking. You can also chew whole pods or steep pods in boiling water for several minutes to make a tea.

Cloves. They pep up digestion and are said to eliminate gas. Add 2 to 3 whole cloves to rice before cooking. Sprinkle on apples and pears when baking. Or steep 2 to 3 whole cloves in a cup of boiling water for ten minutes, sweeten to taste, and drink.

Coriander. This may help in the downward movement of foods being digested and can ease cramps, hiccups, bloating, and flatulence. Crush the seeds into powder and add to foods such as vegetable stir-fry. Its flavor really enhances curry and Middle Eastern dishes, too.

Fennel seeds. It's an acquired taste, but it may be one well worth acquiring if you're plagued by gas. Fennel's digestive powers are so good that in India fennel is customarily eaten after a meal to help digestion and freshen the breath. For gas, drink it as a tea by steeping 1/2 teaspoon seeds in 1 cup boiling water for ten minutes. Or, sprinkle them over those gassy vegetables during cooking or add to stir-fries. If you've acquired the taste, fennel also works well cooked into figs, apples, pears, and plums.

Lemon. Stir 1 teaspoon lemon juice and 1/2 teaspoon baking soda into 1 cup cool water. Drink after meals.

Massage herbs. Add any of these to massage oil and rub over the abdomen to relieve gas: cardamom, clove, cinnamon, fennel, ginger. Warmed olive and sesame oils are wonderful for massages.

Rosemary. If you're eating a gassy food, sprinkle on a little rosemary to cut down the effect. You can do the same with sage and thyme, too.

Tea herbs. Steep and drink a tea made from any of these: aniseed, basil leaves, chamomile, cloves, cinnamon, ginger, peppermint, sage. Steep about 1/2 teaspoon in 1 cup boiling water, then add honey or lemon to taste. Drink one to three times each day.

Turmeric. This may stop a gas problem altogether. Turmeric is one of the many flavorful and curative spices found in curry powder. You can add turmeric itself to rice or season a bland dish with curry powder, which contains turmeric. However you use it, it helps alleviate gas.

Topical Remedies

Heating pad. The warmth of a heating pad placed on your abdomen can help alleviate discomfort.

Pressure. Apply pressure to your abdomen or lie facedown on the floor with a pillow bunched up under your abdomen to help relieve discomfort from gassiness.

Rock and Roll. Sit on the floor with your knees drawn up to your chest and your arms wrapped around your legs, then rock back forth. The pressure and movement may provide relief.

Foot Odor

Foot odor, known in the medical profession as bromhidrosis, can be traced to bacteria that find your moist and warm feet, socks, and shoes the perfect place to breed and multiply. Thousands of sweat glands on the soles of the feet produce perspiration composed of water, sodium chloride, fat, minerals, and various acids that are the end products of your body's metabolism. In the presence of certain bacteria (namely those found in dark, damp shoes), these sweaty secretions break down, generating the stench that turns people green.

Foot odor is only a temporary curse and can easily be cured. Kick off your shoes without worry after trying some of these refreshing remedies.

Topical Remedies

Activated charcoal. Dust some activated charcoal in your shoes. It's an effective (but messy) odor absorbent. Or, you can purchase inexpensive foot pads that contain it.

Baking soda. Don't just let those shoes sit there without odor support. Bring on the baking soda! Deodorize shoes by sprinkling 1 or 2 teaspoons baking soda inside to absorb moisture and hide odors. For added fragrance, combine 3 tablespoons baking soda with 3 tablespoons ground, dried sage leaves. Combine the sage and baking soda and place into an airtight glass jar. After removing your shoes for the day, sprinkle 1 tablespoon of the mixture into each shoe. Shake and leave overnight. The following day, keep the sage-soda in the shoes. In the evening remove excess sage-soda mix, and replace it with a fresh supply. Repeat nightly.

Another way to use baking soda is in a foot bath. Add 2 tablespoons baking soda to a bowl of warm water. Soak feet every night for a month.

Black tea. Soaking your tootsies in black tea will help. Tannic acid, a component of tea, is thought to have astringent properties that prevent feet from perspiring. To make a foot-tea soak, brew 5 bags black tea in 1 quart boiling water. Let cool, add ice cubes (during summertime), and soak in this "iced tea for the toes" bath for 20 to 30 minutes.

Cornstarch. A less fancy solution to keeping shoes deodorized and dry is to sprinkle the inside with 1 to 2 teaspoons cornstarch.

Ginger. Mash a 1- or 2-inch piece of ginger into a pulp, put it into a handkerchief or piece of gauze, and soak it in some hot water for a few minutes. Rub the ginger liquid onto each foot nightly after taking a shower. Try for two weeks.

Radish. You can't squeeze blood from a turnip, but you can squeeze an anti-stink solution from a radish. Using a juice maker, juice about two dozen radishes, add 1/4 teaspoon glycerine, and pour in a squirt or spray-top bottle. Spritz on toes to reduce foot odor.

Salt. Add table salt or Epsom salts to water for a foot soak. Pour a few teaspoons of salt into a tub of warm water. Soak for ten minutes.

Vinegar. Soak your feet several times a week in an apple cider or plain vinegar bath. Mix 1/3 cup vinegar into a bowl of warm water. Soak for 10 to 15 minutes.

Water. A remedy for sweaty feet involves alternating footbaths of hot and cold water to help reduce blood flow to your feet and reduce perspiration. After luxuriating in a hot foot bath, shock those toes by dipping them into a second foot bath containing cool water, ice cubes, and 1 to 2 teaspoons lemon juice (if available). Rub your feet with alcohol following the bath. Try this dual treatment once per day, especially in warmer months.

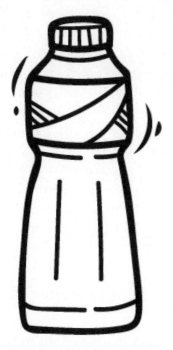

Gout

Gout, which occurs in about five percent of people with arthritis, results from the buildup of uric acid in the blood. Uric acid is the result of the breakdown of waste substances, called purines, in the body. Usually it is dissolved in the blood, processed by the kidneys, and passed out of the body in the urine. But in some people there is an excess amount of uric acid. When there is too much uric acid in the blood, it crystallizes and collects in the joint spaces, causing gout. Occasionally, these deposits become so large that they push against the skin in lumpy patches, called tophi, that can actually be seen.

A gout attack usually lasts five to ten days, and the most common area under siege is the big toe. In fact, 80 percent of people with gout will be affected in the big toe at some time. Gout in the big toe can become so painful that even a bedsheet draped over it will cause intolerable pain. Besides the big toe, gout may also develop in the ankles, heels, knees, wrists, fingers, and elbows.

Though anyone can get gout, it's primarily a man's disease. Women have the good fortune of being more efficient in the way they excrete uric acid. And children rarely get it.

Gout symptoms come on quickly the first time, often overnight. You can go to bed feeling fine and wake up later in excruciating pain. You may also experience joint swelling and shiny red or purple skin around the joint.

If you have gout, professional medical treatment is required. There are several prescription medications that are very effective at eliminating excess uric acid. Untreated, gout may progress to serious joint damage and disability. Also, excess uric acid can cause kidney stones. For gout, though, there are several home remedies that can be effective along with medication to alleviate the pain and symptoms.

Dietary Remedies

Apple preserves. This may neutralize the acid that causes gout. Take as many apples as you wish, then peel, core, and slice. Simmer in a little water for three hours or more, until they turn thick, brown, and sweet. Refrigerate. Use as you would any preserve.

Cherries. Cherries may remove toxins from the body, clean the kidneys, and yes, even help give you a rosy complexion. Because of their cleansing power, they're at the top of the gout-relief list. If you can bake a cherry pie, you may be making a gout treatment. Cherry compote, cherry juice, cherry jam, cherry tea, cherry anything works.

Water. To rid yourself of uric acid, you absolutely must keep your body flushed out. Drink at least 2 quarts of water per day, or more, if you can manage it.

Herbal Remedies

Mustard powder. Make a mustard plaster and apply to the achy joint. Mix 1-part mustard powder (or crushed mustard seeds) to 1 part whole wheat flour and add enough water to form a thick paste. Slather petroleum jelly, vegetable shortening, or lard on the affected area. Spread a thick coat of mustard paste on a piece of gauze or cloth, then apply over the greased-up area. Tape down and leave in place for several hours or overnight.

Thyme. Drink as a tea. Add 1 to 2 teaspoons to a cup of boiling water. Sweeten, if desired, and drink.

Hangovers

Well, you partied from sundown to sunup, and now you're paying the price. You've got the pounding headache, the queasiness, the dizziness, the sensitivity to light and sound, the muscle aches, and the irritability that comes from over-consumption of alcoholic beverages. How quickly last night's fun turns into next morning's nightmare when you have a hangover!

Researchers aren't sure what in the alcohol causes a hangover. But they do know that the debilitating symptoms you experience are a result of the body's inability to get rid of the toxins quickly enough, and they build up in your bloodstream.

The process of metabolizing the alcohol and excreting large quantities of water also robs the body of glucose and other vital nutrients. Being malnourished further contributes to the unpleasant hangover symptoms.

In addition to dehydration, fatigue is also behind some of your hangover pain. Excessive drinking and late nights usually go hand-in-hand. But more than that, alcohol interferes with a normal sleep pattern, robbing you of the dream state, which is essential to feeling rested. You may pass out on the floor and sleep for hours, but it won't be the kind of sleep that will allow you to restart your engines in the morning. Lack of proper rest contributes to the malaise a hangover brings.

The best way to prevent a hangover is, of course, drinking in moderation or abstaining from alcohol. But keeping yourself well-hydrated and well-nourished when you're drinking can go a long way toward minimizing the morning-after symptoms. Try drinking a glass of water or other noncaffeinated beverage for each alcoholic beverage you drink. And don't drink on an empty stomach. Food helps slow the absorption of alcohol, giving your body time to metabolize it and decreasing the chances of a hangover.

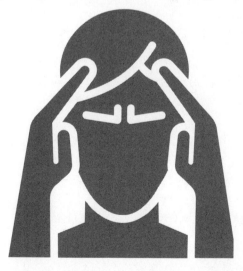

Dietary Remedies

Bananas. While you were drunk and peeing like a racehorse, lots of potassium drained from your body. Eating a banana bursting with potassium will give you some giddy-up and go. All you have to do is peel and eat.

Juice. Juice, especially freshly squeezed orange juice, will help raise your blood sugar levels and help ease some of your hangover symptoms. However, if your stomach is upset, skip acidic juices such as orange juice and stick with apple juice instead.

Rice, soup, or toast. Food is probably the last thing you want to look at while recovering, but you do need some substance for energy. Stay with clear liquids until you can tolerate something solid. Then start off slowly with mild, easy-to-digest foods such as plain toast, rice, or clear soup.

Sports drinks. These are a good way to replace fluids as well as electrolytes and glucose.

Water. Next to time, drinking water is the best cure for a hangover. Dehydration does a doozy on your body and causes much of the discomfort associated with a hangover. Stick to water, be it tap, bottled, or carbonated. Drink more than 8 glasses a day while recovering.

Herbal Remedies

Ginger root. Ginger has long been used to treat nausea and seasickness. And, since having a hangover is much like being seasick, this easy remedy works wonders. If you're really green, the best bet is to drink ginger ale (no preparation required, but be sure to choose a brand that actually contains ginger!). If you can remain vertical for ten minutes, brew some ginger tea. Cut 10 to 12 slices of fresh ginger root and combine with 4 cups water. Boil for ten minutes. Strain and add the juice of 1 orange, the juice of 1/2 lemon, and 1/2 cup honey. Drink to your relief.

Topical Remedies

Ice. Put an ice compress on your aching head. Place crushed iced in a plastic bag, wrap in a dry towel, and apply it to where it hurts. Or just rinse a washcloth under cold water, place it on your forehead, and rest.

Hemorrhoids

Hemorrhoids are a sore subject, and not one that is brought up at the dinner table. Yet privately, millions of people suffer from these painful protrusions. Also known as "piles," hemorrhoids are swollen, stretched out veins that line the anal canal and lower rectum. Internal hemorrhoids may either bulge into the anal canal or protrude out through the anus (these are called prolapsed). External hemorrhoids occur under the surface of the skin near the anal opening. Both types hurt, burn, itch, irritate, and bleed.

About one-half to three-fourths of Americans will develop hemorrhoids in their lifetime. Most cases are caused by constipation or physical strain while making a bowel movement. Other causes include heredity, age, a low fiber diet resulting in constipation, obesity, the improper use of laxatives, pregnancy, anal intercourse, prolonged sitting, and prolonged standing.

Fortunately, most hemorrhoids respond well to home treatments and changes in the diet, so you can keep this sore point under wraps.

Dietary Remedies

Oranges. Vitamin C plays a role in strengthening and toning blood vessels, so eat lots of vitamin C-rich fruits and vegetables.

Prunes. If you haven't eaten a prune since your mother tried to force one down your throat at age five, then it's time to try again. As mama knew, prunes have a laxative effect and help soften stools. Try to eat 1 to 3 per day, and look at it as pleasure, not punishment.

Water. Think of water as the plumber of the digestive tract, without the $85-an-hour fee. Water keeps the digestive process moving along without block-ups—one of the main causes of hemorrhoids. Reaping the benefits requires a minimum of 8 large glasses of water each day. Drinking other fluids, such as juice, and eating plenty of water-loaded fruits and vegetables can help the flow of things.

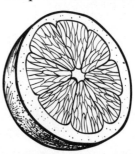

Topical Remedies

Ice. Now here's a remedy guaranteed to wake you up and soothe hemorrhoid pain. Sit on a cold compress. That's right, literally freeze your rear end. Break ice into small cubes (easier for the ice to shape itself around certain regions), and place it in a plastic, reclosable bag. Cover with a thick paper towel and sit on it! The cooling works twofold: First, it numbs the region, and second, it reduces blood flow to those distended veins.

Potato. A poultice made from grated potato works as an astringent and soothes pain. Take 2 washed potatoes, cut them into small chunks, and put them into a blender. Process until the potatoes are in liquid form. Add a few teaspoons water if they look dry. Spread the mashed 'taters into a thin gauze bandage or clean handkerchief, fold in half, and apply to the hemorrhoids for five to ten minutes.

Vinegar. Applying a dab of apple cider or plain vinegar to hemorrhoids stops itching and burning. The vinegar has astringent properties that help shrink swollen blood vessels. After dry wiping, dip a cotton ball in vinegar and apply.

Herbal Remedies

Aloe vera. Versatile aloe vera comes to the rescue once again as a hemorrhoid healer. The very same anti-inflammatory constituents that reduce blistering and inflammation in burns also help reduce the irritation of hemorrhoids. Break off a piece of the aloe vera leaf and apply only the clear gel to the hemorrhoids.

Chamomile. German folk medicine uses chamomile as a hemorrhoid treatment. It contains strong anti-inflammatory substances that may reduce the pain or itching associated with hemorrhoids. To reap the benefits of chamomile, use it in a bath. Combine 1 ounce dried chamomile with 2 quarts boiling water to make a tea. Let steep until warm. Pour the tea into a tub deep enough to sit in and soak for 15 minutes. If possible, bathe two to three times per day for acute hemorrhoids. Or, you can make the tea and apply it to the hemorrhoids with a cotton ball after having a bowel movement. Do not use chamomile if you have pollen allergies.

Hiccups

Even before you were born, you got the hiccups. Just ask your mom. And those strange muscle spasms will continue to come over you for the rest of your days. Everyone gets hiccups. Thankfully most bouts with the hiccups are pretty short-lived, lasting at most a few hours. Hiccups can be somewhat embarrassing, though. Imagine hiccuping through a first date or, worse, making a sales presentation you've worked on for months and letting out a loud "hic" right as you move in for the kill.

One of the physiological reasons experts give for hiccups is an irritation of the nerve that leads from the brain to the abdominal area. Aggravating this nerve starts a chain reaction that touches off the nerve that activates the diaphragm. But what sets the nerve off in the first place?

You get the hiccups for all sorts of reasons. Digestive disturbances, such as eating too fast, eating too much, eating an irritating food, or eating hot and cold foods together, are frequent triggers. Alcohol and fizzy drinks have been blamed for hiccups, and some experts believe they can be caused by emotional stress. But sometimes they occur for no reason. You may be sitting quietly reading a book, when all of a sudden, "hic!" There's no one reason why you get hiccups, and there's no one way to get rid of them!

Most cures involve interrupting your breathing pattern, causing you to take a deep breath or an irregular breath (such as breathing while you swallow). But when you've got the hiccups, you will try almost anything to get rid of them.

Dietary Remedies

Honey. Try swallowing a tablespoon of honey. This overwhelms the mouth with a sweet flavor and may short-circuit the irritated nerve.

Ice. Drink a glass of ice water. A cold drink is believed to shock the system. Or simply apply a piece of ice to the back of the neck. This may shock your body and cause you to take a deep breath.

Lemon. Lemons are believed to overwhelm irritated nerves with a sour taste. This may divert the nerves' attention and get rid of your hiccups.

Pineapple juice. Some think the acidic content of the juice helps stop the hiccups.

Sugar. Experts give a thumbs-up to this remedy. Simply place a spoonful of sugar in your mouth, toward the back of the tongue where sour tastes are tasted. This will enhance the sweet overload you're delivering.

Water. Bartenders swear by this hiccup-relieving trick. Quickly down a glass of water with a spoon in it. The swallowing is probably the reason the hiccups go away, but the spoon seems to take the person's mind off their hiccups. And some people believe gargling with water relieves the hiccups.

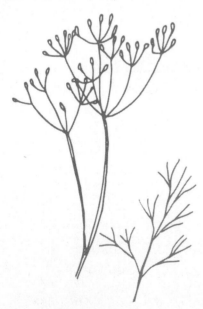

Herbal Remedies

Dill seed. Swallowing a teaspoon of dill seeds is an old folk remedy that may work for you. No one is sure if it's an ingredient in the dill seeds that helps or if simply swallowing the seeds is what does the trick.

Topical Remedies

Cotton swab. Tickling the roof of your mouth with a cotton swab, or your finger, may help cure your hiccups.

Paper bag. Breathing into a paper bag will increase the amount of carbon dioxide in your body. Since your body takes that as a signal of suffocation, your respiratory system urges the body to take deeper breaths. Those deeper breaths may stop the diaphragm spasm. This method is a favorite in hospitals.

Stick 'em up. Putting your hands over your head may help you breathe a bit deeper and lessen the tension on the diaphragm.

Stick it in your ear. Putting your fingers in your ears seems to have some scientific merit in curing hiccups. It works by rerouting the action of the irritated nerve that sparks hiccups. Just be careful not to stick those fingers in too far and cause damage to your inner ear.

Stick out your tongue. Or pull on your tongue. These actions stimulate the glottis and may help keep it open (a closed glottis causes that hiccuping sound) averting your hiccups. Pulling on your tongue also may stimulate your diaphragm and stop its annoying spasms.

Suck it in. Holding your breath works in much the same way that breathing into a paper bag does. It overwhelms your body with carbon dioxide and causes deeper breathing.

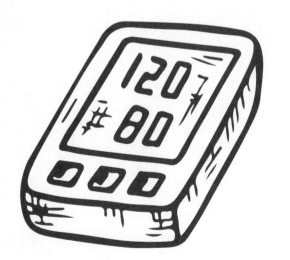

High Blood Pressure

Sometimes what you don't know can hurt you. Such is the case with high blood pressure, or hypertension. Although one in four adults has high blood pressure, according to the American Heart Association (AHA), almost a third of them don't know they have it.

That's because high blood pressure often has no symptoms. It's not as if you feel the pressure of your blood coursing through your circulatory system. When the heart beats, it pumps blood to the arteries, creating pressure within them. That pressure can be normal or it can be excessive. High blood pressure is defined as a persistently elevated pressure of blood within the arteries.

Over time, the excessive force exerted against the arteries damages and scars them. It can also damage organs, such as the heart, kidneys, and brain. High blood pressure can lead to strokes, blindness, kidney failure, and heart failure.

In 90 to 95 percent of all cases, the cause of high blood pressure isn't known. When there is no underlying cause, the disease is known as primary, or essential, hypertension. Sometimes the high blood pressure is caused by another disease, such as an endocrine disorder. In such cases, the disease is called secondary hypertension.

Hypertension is known as "the silent killer" because it has few or no obvious symptoms. The symptoms that it does present are shared by other diseases and conditions. But if you have any of these symptoms, be sure to have your blood pressure checked to rule out high blood pressure:

- Frequent or severe headaches
- Unexplained fatigue
- Dizziness
- Flushing of the face
- Ringing in the ears
- Thumping in the chest
- Frequent nosebleeds

Finding out whether you have high blood pressure is simple. You just need to have your blood pressure checked by a doctor, nurse, or other health professional. Often you can even find blood pressure check booths at your local mall or at the pharmacy. The blood pressure test is simple, quick, and painless, but the results can save your life.

A blood pressure reading is given in two numbers, one over the other. The higher (systolic) number represents the pressure while the heart is beating, indicating how hard your heart has to beat to get that blood moving. The lower (diastolic) number represents the pressure when the heart is resting between beats.

Blood pressure of less than 140 (systolic) over 90 (diastolic) is considered a normal reading for adults, according to the AHA, while a reading equal to or greater than 140 over 90 is considered elevated (high). A systolic pressure of 130 to 139 or a diastolic pressure of 85 to 89 needs to be watched carefully.

The key to controlling high blood pressure is knowing you have it. Under the guidance of a physician, you can battle hypertension through diet, exercise, lifestyle changes, and medication, if necessary. The home holds several blood pressure helpers.

Dietary Remedies

Bananas. The banana has been proved to help reduce blood pressure. The average person needs three to four servings of potassium-rich fruits and vegetables each day. Some experts believe doubling this amount may benefit your blood pressure. If bananas aren't your favorite bunch of fruit, try dried apricots, raisins, currants, orange juice, spinach, boiled potatoes with skin, baked sweet potatoes, cantaloupe, and winter squash.

Breads. Be good to your blood with a bit more "B," as in the B vitamin folate. Swimming around the blood is a substance called homocysteine, which at high levels is thought to reduce the stretching ability of the arteries. If the arteries are stiff as a board, the heart pumps extra hard to move the blood around. Folate helps reduce the levels of homocysteine, in turn helping arteries become pliable. You'll find folate in fortified breads and cereals, asparagus, brussels sprouts, and beans.

Broccoli. This vegetable is high in fiber, and a high fiber diet is known to help reduce blood pressure. Indulge in this and other fruits and vegetables that are high in fiber.

Celery. Because it contains high levels of 3-N-butylphthalide, a phytochemical that helps lower blood pressure, celery is in a class by itself. This phytochemical is not found in most other vegetables. Celery may also reduce stress hormones that constrict blood vessels, so it may be most effective in those whose high blood pressure is the result of mental stress.

Cocoa and chocolate. A 2007 review of 10 studies of chocolate's effects on blood pressure indicated that flavonoid-rich cocoa and chocolate can be part of a blood pressure-lowering diet as long as the total calorie count of the diet stays the same.

Milk. The calcium in milk does more than build strong bones; it plays a modest role in preventing high blood pressure. Be sure to drink skim milk or eat low fat yogurt. Leafy green vegetables also provide calcium.

Polyunsaturated oils. Switching to polyunsaturated oils, such as canola, mustard seed, or safflower, can make a big difference in your blood pressure readings. Switching to them will also reduce your blood cholesterol level.

Herbal Remedies

Cayenne pepper. This fiery spice is a popular home treatment for mild high blood pressure. Cayenne pepper allows smooth blood flow by preventing platelets from clumping together and accumulating in the blood. Add a dash of cayenne to a salad or salt-free soups.

Hives

When you eat a food that you're allergic to, your body reacts by producing histamine. Histamine can do all sorts of things in the body in response to an allergen, such as making your eyes water or your tongue or throat swell. In the case of hives, histamine causes blood vessels to leak blood plasma into the skin. This blood leakage comes to the surface, causing inflammation and itching, and, lucky you, you've got a case of hives.

Hives, whose technical name is urticaria, can be as tiny as a dot or as big as a dinner plate. They have very defined edges and are usually irregularly shaped. If you've ever had hives, you know that though the swelling can be uncomfortable, it's the itching that drives you bonkers. The good news is hives usually run their course in a couple of hours. Sometimes, though, they can last as long as a couple of days. If they last longer than that, you should contact your doctor.

Because hives are an allergic reaction, your best bet in preventing future flare-ups is finding the source of the problem. You'll need to do a little detective work to figure out what caused your itchy bumps. If you can't put your finger on the culprit, you're not alone: About 50 percent of the time the trigger is undetermined.

If you've never had a run-in with the itchy inflammation, you've got a 20 percent chance that you'll end up with it at some point in your life. Young adults are most likely to get hives. Children and adults are at the same risk for getting the itchy red patches, but from different sources. Kids seem to get hives from food allergies or infections, while adults tend to break out in hives in reaction to a medication.

Whether or not you can uncover the source of your hives, there are some home remedies that can help relieve your symptoms while you're investigating.

Herbal Remedies

Asafoetida. This cousin of onions and garlic may help relieve your hives. Look for asafoetida powder in the spice section of your grocery store. Add 1/4 teaspoon asafoetida powder to 4 tablespoons castor oil and mix well. Apply the solution directly to your hives. Be sure to do this when you won't be seeing anyone for a few hours. Asafoetida makes you smell like a piece of garlic.

Basil. The Chinese believe bathing in basil tea is a good antidote for hives. Put 1 ounce dried basil in a 1-quart jar and fill the jar with boiling water. Let cool to room temperature and use it as a wash.

Herbal tea. De-stress yourself by relaxing with a soothing cup of herbal tea.

Topical Remedies

Baking soda. Add 1/2 to 1 cup baking soda to a warm bath to soothe your itching.

Cortisone. An over-the-counter 1 percent topical cortisone preparation may help. Follow the directions on the package.

Cotton gloves or oven mitts. Put these on your hands to keep you from scratching. Tape them at the wrist, and you'll be less tempted to remove them to start scratching. If you wear the gloves to bed at night, you won't do damage if you scratch your itches unconsciously.

Ice. An ice pack helps shrink blood vessels, which alleviates swelling. Put the compress, wrapped in a thin towel, on your skin five minutes at a time, three or four times a day.

Oatmeal. Add 1 to 2 cups finely ground oatmeal to a warm bath (not hot or you might have breakfast for the next month in your tub) to ease your itches.

Milk. Calm your hives with a milk compress. Wet a cloth with cold milk and put it on your skin for 10 to 15 minutes.

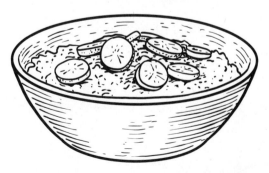

Itching

Itching, medically known as pruritus, is caused by stimuli bugging some part of our skin. There are a lot of places to bother on the body, too. The average adult has 20 square feet of skin, all open to the world of irritants. When something bothers our skin, an itch is a built-in defense mechanism that alerts the body that someone is knocking. We respond to an itch with a scratch, as most people want to remove the problem. But the scratching can also set you up for the "itch-scratch" cycle, where one leads to the other endlessly.

An itch can range from a mild nuisance to a disrupting, damaging, and sleep-depriving fiasco. Itches happen for many reasons, including allergic reactions; sunburns; insect bites; poison ivy; reactions to chemicals, soaps, and detergents; medication; dry weather; skin infections; and even aging. More serious itches, such as those caused by psoriasis or other diseases, are not covered here.

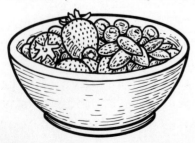

Topical Remedies

Baking soda. Baking soda battles itches of all kinds. For widespread or hard-to-reach itches, soak in a baking soda bath. Add 1 cup baking soda to a tub of warm water. Soak for 30 to 60 minutes and air dry. Localized itches can be treated with a baking soda paste. Mix 3 parts baking soda and 1-part water. Apply to the itch, but do not use if the skin is broken.

Lemon. The aromatic substances in a lemon contain anesthetic and anti-inflammatory properties, which may help reduce itching. If nothing else, you'll smell good. Squeeze undiluted lemon juice on itchy skin and allow to dry.

Oatmeal. Add 1 to 2 cups finely ground oatmeal to a warm, but not hot bath to ease your itches.

Herbal Remedies

Aloe vera. The same constituents that reduce blistering and inflammation in burns also work to reduce itching. Snap off a leaf, slice it down the middle, and rub the gel only on the itch.

Basil. Splash your skin with refreshing basil tea. Like cloves, basil contains high amounts of eugenol, a topical anesthetic. Place 1/2 ounce dried basil leaves in a 1-pint jar of boiling water. Keep it covered to prevent the escape of the aromatic eugenol from the tea. Allow to cool. Dip a clean cloth into the tea and apply to itchy skin as often as necessary.

Mint. If you're saving that basil for spaghetti sauce, try a mint tea rinse instead. Chinese folk medicine values mint as a treatment for itchy skin and hives. Mint contains significant amounts of menthol, which has anesthetic and anti-inflammatory properties when applied topically. To make a mint tea rinse, place 1 ounce dried mint leaves in 1 pint boiling water. Cover and allow to cool. Strain, dip a clean cloth in the tea, and apply to the itchy area when necessary.

Thyme. If you're saving that mint for a glass of lemonade, there is one more spice on the rack that makes a good anti-itch rinse: thyme. This fragrant herb contains large amounts of the volatile constituent thymol, which has anesthetic and anti-inflammatory properties. In other words, it numbs that darn itch while reducing inflammation caused by all your scratching. To make a thyme rinse, place 1/2 ounce dried thyme leaves in a 1-pint jar of boiling water. Cover and allow to cool. Strain and dip a clean cloth into the tea, then apply to affected areas.

Kidney Stones

Each about the size of your fist, your kidneys are located in your back, just below your rib cage. The main function of kidneys is to get rid of extra waste and fluid, clear impurities from the blood, and keep your blood pressure under control. The majority of kidney stones form when there's not enough fluid passing through the kidneys. Certain minerals, namely calcium, magnesium, and phosphate, along with oxalate, a substance found in some foods, begin to crystallize on the sides of the kidneys. When the stones break loose, these little calcified pebbles make a path through your ureter, the tube that connects your kidneys with your bladder. The majority of kidney stones are small, about the size of a tiny pea, and usually pass without notice. Occasionally, however, kidney stones can grow quite large, some even as big as golf balls. As these grainy, rough rounds pass through your ureter, you experience the legendary anguish of passing a stone.

The National Kidney Foundation estimates that one million Americans are treated for kidney stones each year. This doesn't account for the brave souls who pass stones without visiting a doctor. The majority of those with kidney stones will be men, although the number of women with kidney stones is increasing. Experts blame that growing statistic on high protein diets. Too much animal protein in the diet can spark kidney stone formation. Most people have their first attack between ages 20 and 40. And if you have one attack, odds are you'll have another. Fifty percent of people who have kidney stones will have another attack within five years.

If you've ever had a kidney stone, there's some good news. Turns out even those at higher risk for kidney stones can prevent another attack simply by watching what they eat. Here are some suggestions for staying free of kidney stones.

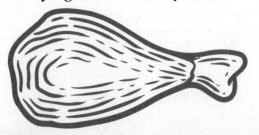

Dietary Remedies

Bran flakes. Fiber helps get rid of calcium and oxalate in your urine, which cuts the risk of kidney stones. A bowl of bran flakes can give you 8 mg of fiber.

Carrots. Vitamin A is an essential ingredient for healthy kidneys. One carrot can give you twice your daily requirements for this kidney-friendly nutrient.

Chicken. The B vitamins, specifically vitamin B6, are well-known stone fighters. Vitamin B6 keeps the body from building up excess oxalate. Too much oxalate is a major factor in kidney stone formation. Three ounces of chicken provide more than one-third of your daily needs.

Milk. Something to put in your strange but true file. Though calcium is one of the major minerals in kidney stones, recent evidence shows that not getting enough calcium can actually increase chances of getting a stone. The reason: When you have lower levels of calcium, your body produces more oxalate, which makes you more at risk for kidney stones. One study found that men who ate the most calcium reduced their chance of developing kidney stones by 34 percent compared with those who ate the least amount of calcium. How much is enough? Meeting your recommended daily allowance, which for most adults is between 1,000 and 1,200 mg a day, the amount in about three glasses of milk, should do the trick.

Tea. Both women and men can benefit from drinking tea. In the Nurses' Health Study, there was an 8 percent decrease in the risk of kidney stones for every 8 ounces of tea the women drank daily. And a Harvard study of men found that there was a 14 percent decrease in kidney stone development for every 8 ounces of tea they drank daily.

Water. Hippocrates was the first person to recognize the benefits of drinking water to averting kidney stones. Most modern-day docs recommend drinking about a gallon of water per day if you're at risk for kidney stones. And drinking fluids at night is more beneficial. If you've never had a stone, stick with the recommended 8 glasses a day.

Whole-wheat bread. A couple slices of whole-wheat bread contain a good amount of magnesium, a mineral known for averting stones. One study found that people who got an adequate

amount of magnesium stopped getting kidney stones altogether.

Menstrual Problems

Ah, that time of the month again. It seems as if it rolls around about every other day, doesn't it? When you were young, anticipating your very first period, you were excited by that passage into womanhood. You didn't anticipate the inconvenience, pain, and all the associated problems: bloat, backache, leg aches, headaches, zits, cramps, and mood swings. And those are on a good menstrual day. On a bad day, bleeding is so heavy you can't move without gushing or you're too tired to breathe. When you figure out that it's more of an inconvenience than something to look forward to, you've joined the true menses sisterhood.

Menstruation is the simple process of shedding the old uterine lining to make way for a new one. In other words, it's the body's way of sweeping out the cobwebs at the end of the month in preparation for the arrival of a new egg and a new cycle; all a part of the natural baby-making process with one goal in mind: conception.

Who experiences menstrual problems? At one time or another, every woman who menstruates. However, some factors make problems more likely.

Most women will experience in the neighborhood of 400 menstrual cycles in their childbearing lifetime. That's a lot of cycles that can cause problems. Serious menstrual problems require medical treatment, since many can lead to infertility, infection, and in some cases, death. But some of the milder problems can be relieved with simple home remedies. And any menstrual relief, no matter how slight, is welcome!

Dietary Remedies

Citrus fruits. Eat or drink with your meals to enhance iron absorption into the body, since iron is easily depleted during menstruation.

Dried apricots. These are high in iron, which is important during menstruation because iron supplies can be depleted with heavy bleeding. Other iron-rich foods are: liver, legumes, shellfish, and fortified breads and cereals.

Red meat. It's loaded with iron as well as zinc, which can be depleted during menses, too. Zinc is necessary for healthy bones, and a zinc deficiency may result in amenorrhea. Other iron- and zinc-rich foods: poultry, fish, green leafy vegetables.

Water. Drink plenty of it. Dehydration can cause the body to produce a hormone called vasopressin that contributes to cramps.

Dietary Supplement Remedies

Vitamin K. Women who have heavy periods may find relief by taking vitamin K supplements. This is the case even if the blood levels of the vitamin are within the normal range. If you take blood-thinning medication such as Coumadin, talk with our doctor before increasing or decreasing your vitamin K intake.

Herbal Remedies

Basil. This can relieve some of the normal pain associated with menstruation because it contains caffeic acid, which has an analgesic, or pain-killing, effect. Thyme is also high in caffeic acid. Use it as a spice in cooking meat and vegetables or Italian dishes. Or steep the herb into tea, adding 2 tablespoons thyme or basil leaves to 1 pint boiling water. Cover tightly and let cool to room temperature. Drink 1/2 to 1 cup an hour for painful menstruation.

Chamomile. This is known to be a reliable cramp reliever. Place 1/2 ounce in a 1-pint jar and cover with boiling water. Steep for one hour, strain, and drink a cup every hour or two. Use honey to sweeten to taste. This is a particularly relaxing tea just before bed.

Cinnamon. This has anti-inflammatory and antispasmodic properties that relieve cramps. Use as a tea, or sprinkle on toast or sweet rolls. If you have a heavy period, drinking cinnamon tea the day before or during your period may help.

Fennel. Another cramp cure, this spice promotes better circulation to the ovaries. Crush 1 teaspoon fennel seeds into a powder. Add to 1 cup boiling water, steep five minutes, strain, and drink hot.

Ginger. This is a cramp reliever, and as an added bonus it some-

times can make irregular periods regular. Use in cookies, cake, and candy or as a spice in vegetables and stir-fries. Tea may be the most effective form, however: put 1/2 teaspoon in 1 cup boiling water, and drink three times per day.

Juniper berries. Steeped into a tea, this can bring on delayed menstruation. Crush 1 teaspoon juniper berries in a coffee grinder or food processor. Place 1 teaspoon of the powder into a cup and fill with boiling water. Steep ten minutes, then take 1/4 cup doses every three to four hours. Do not take this tea if you have kidney disease, or for more than three weeks.

Warning! Juniper berries can trigger preterm birth, so avoid if you may be pregnant.

Lemon balm. This is another cramp reliever, also used for menstruation delayed by stress and tension. Lemon balm also has a mild sedative effect. Make the tea by placing 1 ounce of the herb in 1 quart boiling water, then letting it cool to room temperature. Strain and drink 1/2 cup per hour until the cramps are gone.

Mint. Either peppermint or wintergreen can relieve cramps. Steep into a tea and drink a cup or two per day. Try sucking on mint candy, too.

Motherwort. This herb has a folk use in curing menstrual cramps and delayed menstruation, and it has sedative properties that can relieve stress or nervousness. Place 1/2 ounce of the dried flowering tops in a 1-pint jar and cover with boiling water. Let stand for 20 minutes, then strain and rebottle. Take 1 to 2 ounces of the tea every two to three hours for up to three days. Do not use if you are taking a medication for a thyroid or heart condition, or if menstrual bleeding is heavy.

Mustard. A tablespoon or two of powdered mustard in a basin of nice warm water can relieve cramps, but don't drink it. Soak your feet in it to reap the relaxing effects.

Raspberry leaf. This is an old Native American cure for cramps, used by the Chippewa, Cherokee, Iroquois, Kwakiutl, and Quinalt tribes. Place 1 ounce raspberry leaf in 1 pint water, then bring to a slow boil. Cover and simmer on the lowest heat 30 to 40 minutes. Cool, stir, strain, bottle. Sweeten to taste. One raspberry leaf contains: 408 mg calcium, 446 mg potassium, 106 mg magnesium, 4 mg manganese, and 3.3 mg iron.

Yarrow. A tea made with this herb can stop excessive or prolonged bleeding. It can be taken during the period for bleeding relief or at the beginning to make the entire period easier.

Topical Remedies

Hot water. Put it in a hot water bottle and place on the abdomen to relieve cramps. Or soak a kitchen towel, then wring out excess water, heat in microwave for a minute, and place on abdomen. Be careful not to burn yourself.

Motion Sickness

Modern transportation hasn't eliminated motion sickness (an affliction caused when the eyes and inner ears send conflicting sensory information to the brain). Anyone who has experienced motion sickness would agree that it is a horrible feeling.

No one can completely avoid motion sickness. Even astronauts have bouts of nausea every now and then. For most people, motion sickness comes on fairly quickly and usually involves one of these symptoms: sweating, hyperventilation, dizziness, paleness, the sensation of spinning, loss of appetite, and of course, nausea.

However, you don't have to reach for medication to ward off that queasiness before you take to the road, skies, or seas.

Dietary Remedies

Apple juice. Drink a glass of apple juice with your pre-travel low fat meal. Giving your body a bit of sugar with fluids before you start your journey should help you down the road. And if you start feeling ill, sipping (not gulping) some juice may help you feel better. Almost any non-citrus juice will do. Citrus juice irritates an already unstable stomach.

Crackers. Take these easily digestible snacks along and nibble on them every couple of hours to help prevent nausea and vomiting. An empty stomach makes it more likely that you will get sick.

Ice. Sucking on some ice chips may help calm your stomach and help divert your attention from your unsettled tummy.

Low fat foods. If you eat a low-fat meal before you head out on your trip, you may avoid getting sick. Eating something before you leave makes your stomach more capable of handling the ups and downs of the road. Experts say not eating destabilizes the stomach's electrical signals, making you susceptible to nausea and vomiting.

Peppermint candies or lozenges. If you start feeling sick, get out the peppermints. Not only will you end up with fresh minty breath when you arrive at your destination, you'll also calm your queasiness. And if you're traveling with little ones, try placing 1 drop peppermint oil on their tongues before the trip.

Tea. Sip on some warm tea if you start feeling sick. Warm beverages tend to be easier on a nauseated tummy than a tall glass of cold water. Go for the decaf brew; caffeinated drinks aren't a good idea for unstable stomachs.

Herbal Remedies

Ginger. Ginger has long been an herbal remedy for queasiness, but modern science has proved this spice has merit, especially for motion sickness. One study discovered that ginger was actually better than over-the-counter motion sickness drugs. Make a ginger tea to take along with you when you're traveling by cutting 10 to 12 slices of fresh ginger and placing them in a pot with 1 quart water. Boil for ten minutes. Strain out the ginger, and add 1/2 cup honey or maple syrup for sweetening if you like.

Nausea and Vomiting

It happens to everybody. No one gets a free pass. But that doesn't make the misery of nausea and vomiting any easier on your system.

Nausea is a warning signal; it means stop eating, let your stomach rest. Vomiting is a warning signal, too; it means something doesn't belong in your stomach and it's time to get rid of it. In other words, nausea and vomiting are two ways that your tummy protects itself.

Although your first inclination after vomiting is to find some way to stop it from happening again, this emetic rush is really your friend because it often does get rid of whatever is ailing you. On occasion, however, nausea and vomiting drag

on. You may be able to cope with ongoing nausea, but there are risks to repeated vomiting. If you vomit a lot or for many days, you can become dehydrated quickly. And if vomiting accompanies morning sickness, the nutritional flow to the developing fetus may be impaired.

Because nausea and vomiting are usually just sideshows and not the main event, under most circumstances they can be remedied right in your home without too much fuss or muss. Here are several ways to put them in their place.

Dietary Remedies

Cranberry juice. Avoiding solid food for a day is sometimes recommended when you're nauseated and vomiting, but don't give up the fluids. Drink cranberry juice during your fast. It's generally easy on your digestive tract.

Lemon juice. Mix together 1 teaspoon honey and 1 teaspoon lemon juice. And this cure comes with a folkish instruction: Dip your finger into the mix and lick it off so that you take it in slowly.

Lime juice. For an immediate nausea/vomiting stopper, mix 1 cup water, 10 drops lime juice, and 1/2 teaspoon sugar. Then add 1/4 teaspoon baking soda and drink.

Milk. Don't drink it straight. Instead, try this vintage milk toast recipe for a bland food that's easy to eat when combating nausea and vomiting. Heat 1 cup milk until hot but not boiling. Put it in a bowl. Then take 1 piece of toast, slightly buttered, and crumble it into the milk. Eat slowly.

Onion. Juice an onion to make 1 teaspoon. Mix with 1 teaspoon grated ginger and take for nausea.

Peppermint candy. Peppermint anesthetizes the stomach, which reduces the gag reflex and stops vomiting. Suck on a piece or two to rid yourself of the symptoms.

Popcorn. Air pop a cup or two and place in a bowl. Do not add butter or salt. Instead, pour enough boiling water over the popcorn to cover it, then let it stand for 15 minutes. Popcorn is a carbohydrate that's especially necessary if you've been vomiting or skipping meals, and the added water is good for dehydration.

Salt. Mix together 1 heaping teaspoon salt, 1 heaping teaspoon red pepper, and 1 cup

vinegar. Take 1 tablespoon every half hour, as needed.

Soda crackers. Chewing on a few of these can help quell nausea.

Vinegar. To stop the nausea of morning sickness, stir 1 teaspoon apple cider vinegar into 1 glass water and drink.

Herbal Remedies

Aniseed. This helps cure nausea and vomiting. Brew aniseed into a tea by putting 1/4 teaspoon in 1/2 cup boiling water. Steep for five minutes. Strain and drink once per day. Or sprinkle some aniseed on mild vegetables such as carrots or pumpkin. If your stomach will tolerate fruits during or just after a bout of nausea or vomiting, try aniseed on baked apples or pears.

Cinnamon. Steep 1/2 teaspoon cinnamon powder in 1 cup boiling water, strain, and sip for nausea. Do not try this remedy if you're pregnant.

Clove. This makes a nice nausea-fighting tea. Brew a cup using 1 teaspoon clove powder in a teacup full of boiling water. Strain out any clove that might be remaining, and drink as needed.

Cumin. Steep a tea with 1 teaspoon cumin seeds and a pinch of nutmeg to soothe tummy troubles.

Fennel. Crush 1 tablespoon seeds and steep for ten minutes in 1 cup boiling water. Sweeten to taste with honey. Sip as necessary for nausea.

Ginger. Without a doubt, ginger is the best stomach woe cure of all. Taken in any form, it will relieve nausea. Try ginger tea, gingerbread, or gingersnaps. If you're traveling, take along ginger sticks or crystallized ginger instead of travel sickness pills or patches. Studies show ginger to be more effective than the potion you purchase at the pharmacy. Skip the ginger ales, though, unless they have real ginger content. Much of today's ginger ale is absent its curative ginger.

Mint. Mint tea relieves nausea. Simply steep about 1 tablespoon dry leaves in 1 pint hot water for 30 minutes; strain and drink. Don't toss out those mint leaves when you drink the tea. Instead, eat them. Eating boiled mint leaves can cure nausea, too.

Topical Remedies

Try a cold compress. Draping a cold compress on your head can be very comforting when you're vomiting.

Nosebleeds

Nosebleeds can run the gamut from a tiny trickle to a big gush. It may be disturbing to see blood drip from your otherwise placid nose, but there is usually no need to worry. Nosebleeds are typically harmless annoyances. It may look like you're losing lots of blood, but the amount is usually insignificant.

The inner nose is one of the more sensitive parts of the body. Lined with hundreds of blood vessels that reside close to the surface, the nostrils don't take kindly to being harassed and will bleed with little provocation, which can come from a number of sources.

The main way to stop a nosebleed is to firmly but gently pinch your nostrils closed, holding them tightly together for at least ten minutes. Lean forward to prevent blood from running down the throat. In addition to this first line of treatment, there are other means to help stop a nosebleed as well as prevent one.

Dietary Remedies

Dark green leafy vegetables. These are high in vitamin K, which is essential for proper blood clotting.

Oranges and orange juice. Keeping those blood vessels in top form is one way to prevent them from breaking so easily. Vitamin C is necessary to the formation of collagen, which helps create a moist lining in your nose. Drink and eat vitamin C-rich foods to help stave off nosebleeds.

Water. Dry winter air and mountain air can dry out the nose in no time. Being well hydrated helps. Always drink 8 glasses of water per day, but have a few more during the driest times and in the driest places.

Whole-wheat bread. Zinc is a nutrient known to help maintain the body's blood vessels. Eat whole-wheat bread and brown rice, two foods high in zinc. Or, for a snack, try some popcorn, which also contains zinc.

Topical Remedies

Baking soda. Used for nasal irrigation and to treat dryness.

Ice. Ice is nice for stopping bleeding, constricting the blood vessels, and reducing inflammation (if the nose is injured). Place crushed iced into a plastic zipper-type bag and cover with a towel. (A bag of frozen vegetables works fine, too.) Place the compress on the bridge of the nose and hold until well after the bleeding stops.

Salt. Nasal irrigation, commonly used by allergy sufferers to rid the nasal passages of mucus, dust, and other gunk, also helps soothe and moisturize irritated nasal membranes. You'll need 1 to 1 1/2 cups lukewarm water (do not use softened water), a bulb (ear) syringe (typically found with baby products in the pharmacy), 1/4 to 1/2 teaspoon salt, and 1/4 to 1/2 teaspoon baking soda. Mix the salt and baking soda into the water, and test the temperature. To administer, suck in the water using the bulb and squirt the saline solution into one nostril while holding the other closed. Lower your head over the sink and gently blow out the water. Repeat this, alternating nostrils until the water is gone. You can also buy a neti pot, a device used to accomplish the irrigation, at drugstores.

Steam. Take every opportunity to breathe steam, be it from your morning tea or from a mini steam bath. To do the latter, boil 1/2 pot water and put on a sturdy surface. Place a towel over your head, lean forward, and breathe gently. Don't lean in too far or you'll burn your sniffer! Try a mini steam bath twice a day.

Vinegar. Take a cloth or cotton ball and wet it with white vinegar. Plug it in the nostril that's bleeding. Vinegar helps seal up the blood vessel wall.

Dietary Supplement Remedies

Vitamin E. Keep your nasal membranes moisturized by applying vitamin E several times a day. Break open a capsule and coat your pinky finger or a cotton swab and gently wipe it just inside your nostrils. This is especially good to do at night before going to sleep.

Osteoporosis

More than 34 million Americans are at risk for osteoporosis, and more than 10 million already have been diagnosed with this bone-degenerating disease. Women make up an astounding 80 percent of those who are affected by osteoporosis. Though most people associate osteoporosis with older people, the disease strikes young and old alike. Osteoporosis does become much more common as you age, affecting one in two women over age 50.

Osteoporosis literally means porous bones. That means someone diagnosed with the disease has lost so much density that there's not much there to hold their bones together, putting them at greater risk for bone breaks and fractures. The National Osteoporosis Foundation calls osteoporosis the "silent disease" because there are virtually no symptoms of bone loss. Unless you're aware of the risk factors and take action, you may not know you have the disease until some benign bump on the garage door turns into a fracture.

One of the greatest risk factors for osteoporosis is something you can't see and you can't control, heredity. Other risk factors include:

not getting enough calcium, having an eating disorder, using certain medications such as corticosteroids, not exercising, and smoking.

Thankfully, there are many ways you can combat and even reverse the damaging effects of this bone-thinning disease, and the earlier you start the better. Why not try some of the bone boosters in your home?

Dietary Remedies

Apples. Boron is a trace mineral that helps your body hold on to calcium, the building block of bones. It even acts as a mild estrogen replacement, and losing estrogen is instrumental in speeding bone loss. Boron is found in apples and other fruits such as pears, grapes, dates, raisins, and peaches. It's also in nuts such as almonds, peanuts, and hazelnuts.

Bananas. Eat a banana a day to build your bones. Studies have found that women who have diets high in potassium also have stronger bones in their spines and hips. Researchers think this is related to potassium's ability to keep blood healthy and balanced so the body doesn't have to suck calcium from the skeleton to keep blood up to par.

Broccoli. Eat 1/2 cup broccoli to get your daily dose of vitamin K. Studies are finding that postmenopausal women with low levels of this vital vitamin are more likely to have osteoporosis.

Margarine. Slather a teaspoon of low trans fatty margarine on your toast for a dose of vitamin D. Vitamin D helps the body absorb calcium, a necessary ingredient to bone health.

Milk. When it comes to strong bones, getting enough calcium is a must. One cup of milk can provide 300 mg of the 1,000 to 1,200 mg of calcium the government recommends you get every day.

Orange juice. Grab a glass of OJ to get your vitamin C. Necessary for the body processes that rebuild bones, getting enough vitamin C is vital to preventing osteoporosis. Grab some calcium-fortified orange juice and get a healthy dose of bone-building nutrients.

Peanut butter. A recent review of studies on nutrition and osteoporosis found that magnesium was a vital component to strengthening, preserving, and rebuilding bones. You can get 50 mg of magnesium by eating 2 tablespoons of peanut butter.

Pineapple juice. Drink a cup of pineapple juice and give your body some manganese. Studies are finding that manganese deficiency is a predictor of osteoporosis. Other manganese sources are oatmeal, nuts, beans, cereals, spinach, and tea.

Tofu. Soy is showing promise as a potential bone strengthener. Soy contains proteins that act like a weak estrogen in the body. These "phytoestrogens," or plant-based estrogens, may help women regain bone strength.

Dietary Supplement Remedies

Calcium. If you don't get enough calcium in your diet, be sure to use a supplement to help prevent osteoporosis.

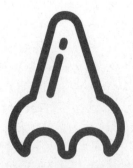

Postnasal Drip

You may wake up with a sore throat, a hacking cough, or simply clearing your throat every morning, or you may just feel as if something has settled in the back of your throat. Any of those experiences could mean that you've got postnasal drip.

On any given day, you've got one to two quarts of mucus running down the back of your throat. That's an awful lot of slime running through your head, but it serves a significant purpose. Mucus acts as a broom, cleaning out the nasal passages. It kicks out bacteria, viruses, and other infection-causing invaders and clears out other foreign particles. Mucus also helps humidify the air that travels in your body, keeping you and your insides comfortable. Unless you think about it, you probably don't even notice all that mucus making its way down your throat. But if you become acutely aware of mucus in the back of your throat, or feel as if someone has turned on a faucet in your head, you're probably dealing with postnasal drip.

Postnasal drip happens when mucus production goes awry. There may be an overproduction of mucus, which gives you that typical drip, drip, drip feeling in the back of your throat. The mucus is clear, thin, and very runny. At the other extreme is thick, sticky mucus that is yellow or green. This kind of mucus occurs when mucus production slows down and thickens, hanging around in the throat.

Most problems with postnasal drip are merely irritating and eventually will go away. But you can alleviate some symptoms with home remedies.

Dietary Remedies

Water. Drinking enough water is a commonsense defense against postnasal drip. It keeps your mucus thin and your body, including your nasal passages, well hydrated. Drink at least eight 8-ounce glasses of water a day.

Topical Remedies

Baking soda. If you're willing to do anything to clear up your mucus problem, try this remedy. Mix 1 cup warm water, 1 teaspoon salt, and a pinch of baking soda. Get a nasal syringe and squirt the mixture into your nostril, closing off

the back of your palate and your throat. Tilt your head back, forward, and to each side for eight to ten seconds in each position to get the solution through all four of your sinus cavities. After you swish everything around, blow your nose. Try squirting in three or four bulbs full of the solution on each side of your nose. If you don't have a bulb syringe, you can snort the mixture out of your cupped hand. Try this process up to six times per day when you're dealing with postnasal drip. If you want to avoid future problems, do it twice per day.

Salt. Gargling with salt water can help soothe your sore throat. Add 1/2 teaspoon salt to 1 cup water and gargle away.

Poor Appetite

A poor appetite can stem from many factors. Perhaps the most common causes are emotional upset, nervousness, tension, anxiety, or depression. Stressful events, such as losing a job or a death in the family, can also make the appetite plummet. Diseases such as influenza and acute infections play a role in appetite reduction, as do anorexia nervosa and fatigue. Illegal and legal drugs, including amphetamines, antibiotics, cough and cold medications, codeine, and morphine can also take a toll on the appetite. Sometimes poor eating habits, such as continuous snacking, can lead to a poor appetite at mealtimes. A poor appetite can also be one symptom of a serious disease.

Fortunately, for minor cases of poor appetite, the kitchen is the best place to get the appetite back into gear.

breaking them apart for absorption. This is important because fats carry essential fatty acids, such as heart-healthy omega-3s, along with fat-soluble vitamins A, D, E, and K and carotenoids such as beta-carotene.

Water. The wonders of water never cease. Water helps control the appetite, especially when you drink the recommended daily amount: 8 glasses! Don't skimp, even if you don't feel like drinking.

Dietary Remedies

Bitter greens. Mama always told you to eat your greens. If she knew you weren't eating properly, she might add, eat your "bitter" greens. Bitter greens consist of arugula, radicchio, collards, kale, endives, escarole, mizuna, sorrel, dandelions, watercress, and red/green mustard...in other words, all those leaves you find in fancy restaurant salads. Stimulating digestion is the name of the game with bitter greens. They prompt the body to make more digestive juices and digestive enzymes. Bitter foods also stimulate the gallbladder to contract and release bile, which helps break fatty foods into small enough particles that enzymes can easily finish

Herbal Remedies

Caraway. The early Greeks knew caraway could calm an upset stomach and used it to season foods that were hard to digest. Today, unsuspecting cooks who simply love the flavor of caraway continue the tradition by adding caraway to rye bread, cabbage dishes, sauerkraut and coleslaw, pork, cheese sauces, cream soups, goose, and duck. One of the easiest ways to enjoy caraway is with a good helping of sauerkraut. Sauté 1/2 medium onion in 1 to 2 tablespoons butter. When onions turn deep golden brown, add 1 can sauerkraut and its liquid along with 1 or 2 tablespoons brown sugar and 1 teaspoon caraway seeds. Let the mixture simmer (covered) for 1 hour. Serve as a side dish with meat, poultry, or sausage.

Cayenne pepper. Nothing revs up the old digestive engine like cayenne. Cayenne pepper has the power to make any dish fiery hot, but it also has a subtle flavor-enhancing quality. There is some evidence that eating hot pepper increases metabolism and the appetite. Add a few shakes of cayenne pepper to potato salad, deviled eggs, chili, and other hot dishes such as stews and soups.

Fennel. Fennel, like its cousin caraway (both belong to the Umbelliferae family of herbs), is a familiar digestive aid, both for relieving stomach upset and for boosting the appetite.

Ginger. Ginger helps stimulate a tired appetite, both through its medicinal properties and its refreshing taste. Try nibbling on gingersnaps or sipping ginger ale made with real ginger. Ginger tea is also a way to start the day off on an appetizing note. To make, place 1/2 teaspoon powdered ginger into a cup and fill with boiling water. Cover and let stand ten minutes. Strain and sip. Don't take more than three times daily. If needed, sweeten with just a little honey. Warning!

Pregnant women should consult a doctor before taking ginger.

Mint. Peppermint refreshes the palate and revives the appetite. Make a cup of mint tea and enjoy anytime you don't feel like eating. Place 1 tablespoon mint leaves in a 1-pint jar of boiling water. Let stand 20 to 30 minutes, shaking occasionally. Strain and sip as needed. If you're tired of teas, make a glass of mint lemonade by adding a few sprigs to the lemonade mixture and letting it sit for ten minutes before sipping.

Premenstrual Syndrome

It's that soon-to-be-time of the month, and all of a sudden you do the Jekyll-Hyde switch. Your mild, calm demeanor is replaced by rages, and your emotions become unstable. Sometimes you feel out of control. At this time of the month, friends and loved ones may do their best to avoid you.

These mood swings, along with a host of other symptoms such as water retention, breast swelling and tenderness, depression, irritability, fatigue, food cravings, and headaches, are known as premenstrual syndrome (PMS). They typically begin a few days to a week before menstruation and end when the menstrual period begins.

Researchers believe that about 40 percent of women of child-bearing age experience PMS in some form. Symptoms and severity vary from mild and manageable to severe and disruptive. Some women only have one symptom, while others have a whole constellation of problems. PMS can be downright brutal for about 15 percent of women who experience many symptoms to a debilitating degree, causing serious problems on the job and in interpersonal relationships.

Even though it's not fully understood, PMS is now recognized as a legitimate condition, not something that's all in women's heads. There are medications available that can mitigate or stop many of the harshest symptoms. Like so many other conditions, though, there are simple home treatments that can work in relieving symptoms. If you're a PMS sufferer, you know that anything that might help is worth a try.

Dietary Remedies

Avocados. These contain natural serotonin, which may supplement the mood-lifting brain chemical naturally produced by the body. Dates, plums, eggplants, papayas, plantains, and pineapple are also sources of serotonin.

Bananas. Rich in potassium, they can relieve the bloating and swelling of water retention that comes with PMS. Other foods such as figs, black currants, potatoes, broccoli, onions, and tomatoes are potassium-rich, too.

Cherries. An Ayurvedic remedy to relieve PMS symptoms, including bloating and mood swings, is to eat 10 fresh cherries on an empty stomach each day for one week before the start of the menstrual period.

Chicken. It's rich in Vitamin B6, which may be depleted in women who suffer from PMS. Vitamin B6 may help relieve depression by raising levels of serotonin, a mood-enhancer, in the brain. Other B6-rich foods include fish, milk, brown rice, whole grains, soybeans, beans, walnuts, and green leafy vegetables.

Oatmeal. It breaks down slowly and gradually releases sugar into the bloodstream. This slow, steady release combats the cravings that come with PMS. Rye bread, pasta, basmati rice, and fruit produce the same effect.

Pasta. This is enriched with magnesium, which is important for normal hormonal function. A lack of magnesium may be the cause of muscle cramps. Other magnesium-rich foods include green vegetables, breakfast cereals (skip those sugary ones), and potatoes.

Sunflower seeds. They're rich in omega-6 fatty acid, which may be missing in women who suffer with PMS. Pumpkin and sesame seeds are also loaded with it.

Turkey. It supplies tryptophan, an amino acid that converts into serotonin, a mood-enhancer. Cottage cheese is another source of tryptophan.

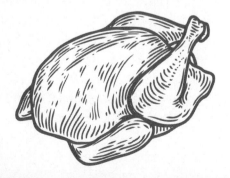

Herbal Remedies

Black pepper. Add a pinch to 1 tablespoon aloe vera gel, and take three times per day with meals to relieve symptoms such as backache and abdominal pain. Aloe vera gel taken with a pinch of cumin works well, too.

Chasteberry. This PMS herb has a reputation among herbalists as one of the best PMS symptom-beaters. As an extract, put 15 drops under your tongue, twice per day. As a tea, add 1 tablespoon chasteberry and 3 tablespoons red raspberry leaves to 1 quart boiling water. Steep 20 minutes, strain, and drink 2 cups per day.

Cinnamon. Good sleep habits are important in the treatment of PMS, and a brew of cinnamon tea is relaxing just before bed. Sweeten to taste with honey. Chamomile tea is a relaxing bedtime choice, too.

Evening primrose oil. This is beginning to get recognition from traditional medical sources as a powerful PMS reliever. Take 3,000 mg per day, in divided doses. Begin taking it ten days before your period is expected to start.

Rose petals. A simple tea of fresh or dried petals may cure irritability or agitation. Simply steep a few in 1 cup boiling water. Petals can be added to fruit and vegetable salads, too.

Topical Remedies

Ice. If you're suffering tension or extreme anxiety, a nice cooling drink may be relaxing. Or wrap some ice in a kitchen towel to use as a cold compress on aching muscles and PMS headaches.

Kitchen towel. Soak it in water, wring it out, then warm it up in the microwave for a minute. Moist heat is soothing, so apply this to your belly when you're having abdominal or ovarian cramps. Be careful not to burn yourself.

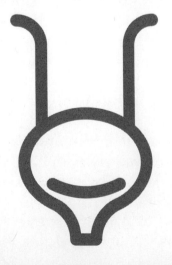

Prostate Problems

It's a sad fact of growing older for the male species: Most men older than 60 (and some in their 50s) develop some symptoms of prostate problems. The three most common disorders are benign prostatic hyperplasia (BPH), a noncancerous enlargement of the prostate; prostatitis, an inflammatory infection; and prostate cancer. BPH is so common that some physicians consider it a normal consequence of aging in males.

The prostate's main role is to produce an essential portion of the seminal fluid that carries sperm. This walnut-shaped gland located just below a man's bladder starts to kick in near puberty and continues to grow. This enlargement doesn't usually cause symptoms until after age 40, and it usually doesn't cause problems until age 60 or later.

An enlarged prostate is problematic because it presses on the urethra, creating difficulties with urination and weakening the bladder. Ignoring prostate problems, as some men are wont to do, isn't a smart idea. Left untreated, prostate problems can get progressively worse, become more painful, and can lead to dangerous complications, including bladder and kidney infections.

Changes in diet can help relieve some prostate discomforts and, in some cases, may reduce the chances of developing prostate cancer.

Dietary Remedies

Corn silk. The silk from corn has been used by Amish men for generations as a remedy for the symptoms of prostate enlargement. When fresh corn is in season, cut the silk from 6 ears of corn. (Corn silk can be dried for later use, too.) Put in 1 quart water, boil, and simmer for ten minutes. Strain and drink a cup. Drink 3 cups per week.

Fish. From the deep comes a way to fight prostate cancer and tumor growth. Try to get 2 servings per week of fish high in omega-3 oils (the good oil) such as tuna, mackerel, or salmon.

Pumpkin seeds. Pumpkin seeds are used by German doctors to treat difficult urination that accompanies an enlarged prostate that is not cancerous. The seeds contain diuretic properties and plenty of zinc, which helps repair and build the immune system. The tastiest way to enjoy pumpkin seeds is to eat them plain. Remove the shells and don't add salt. You can also try a tea. Crush a handful of fresh seeds and place in the bottom of a 1-pint jar. Fill with boiling water. Let cool to room temperature. Strain and drink a pint of pumpkin seed tea per day.

Soy. Learning to like and use soy foods is an easy and good way to help nip prostate problems in the bud. Soy-based foods contain phytoestrogens, which are thought to help reduce testosterone production, which is believed to aggravate prostate cancer growth. The phytoestrogens are believed to limit the growth of blood capillaries that form around tumors of the prostate.

Tomatoes. Seize that salsa! Pour on the spaghetti sauce! Down that tomato juice! Learn to add more tomatoes to your diet. Studies have shown that as little as 2 servings of tomatoes (including cooked tomatoes) per week can help men reduce their risk of prostate cancer by half. These red orbs are full of lycopene, an antioxidant compound that helps fight cancer.

Watermelon seeds. The Amish use watermelon tea to flush the system out and help with bladder problems and prostate problems. Enjoy a slice of watermelon and spit the seeds in a cup. When you have 1/8 cup fresh watermelon seeds, put them in a 1-pint jar and fill with boiling water. Let the tea cool, strain, and drink. Drink 1 pint of tea every day for ten days.

Dietary Supplement Remedies

Saw palmetto. The extract of the berries of this plant has been shown to work as well or better than prescription drugs in improving urinary flow rates and reducing the symptoms of BPH, such as urinary hesitancy and weak flow. The extract works by altering certain hormone levels, thus reducing prostate enlargement. Palmetto extracts can be purchased at the health food store. Consult your physician for recommended dosages.

Stinging nettle. Stinging nettle has been used in Europe for more than a decade, and studies have shown it to reduce symptoms of prostate problems. Nettle helps by inhibiting binding of testosterone-related proteins to their receptor sites on prostate cell membranes. Take stinging nettle in extract form (as

capsules). Check with your physician for the correct dosage.

Seasonal Affective Disorder

Ho hum. Another day, so much to do. But you can't seem to drag yourself out of bed. If that's a description of the way you feel every winter, you could be suffering from seasonal affective disorder, or SAD. It's a poorly understood condition that affects some people during the winter months when there is less sunlight.

In addition to a depressed mood, symptoms of SAD include cravings for carbohydrates, inability to concentrate, irritability, lethargy, weight gain, and a lack of interest in sex.

Although the link between the gray, short days of winter and SAD is well-established, no one knows why some people are affected and others are not. Current thinking associates SAD with too much melatonin, the hormone that causes you to be sleepy. Normally, sunlight stops melatonin production in the body, and darkness starts it. When adequate sunlight is missing, as it usually is in the winter months, that wanna-go-to-sleep hormone kicks into overtime production because there's nothing around to tell it to turn itself off.

Some medical researchers compare SAD to hibernation. During the winter, many animals store up on the carbohydrates, crawl into a cozy cave, resist the mating urge, and snooze until spring. Sounds pretty primal, but that's exactly the way people who suffer SAD react, only in a modified version.

Another theory is that SAD is a result of a delay in the timing of the body clock. In SAD patients, the body's lowest temperature occurs at 6 A.M., rather than at 3 A.M., as it should normally. As a result, they are awakening when physiologically it is the middle of the night. When treated with light from 6 A.M. to 8 A.M., these patients experience a shift in minimum temperature to an earlier time and an associated shift in mood.

Doctors often treat SAD with antidepressants. For some, they work. For others, the side effects are overwhelming, often worse than the SAD itself.

Dietary Remedies

Apricots. This fruit gradually raises serotonin levels and helps keep them there, as do apples, pears, grapes, plums, grapefruits, and oranges.

Avocados. They are high in natural serotonin, which seems to suppress appetite. Also high in natural serotonin are dates, bananas, plums, eggplant, papayas, passion fruit, plantains, pineapples, and tomatoes.

Basmati rice. The sugar in this rice is slow to release into the bloodstream, which helps blood sugar levels stay constant instead of going through highs and lows. Drastic changes in blood sugar can lead to weight gain, which is a side effect of SAD. Other foods with a similar effect on blood sugar are rye bread and pasta.

Bouillon. When the carbohydrate craving is just about to defeat you, drink some hot bouillon or broth. Hot liquids in the belly are filling, and consuming them before a meal is an old diet trick that reduces food consumption. Better the bouillon than the banana cream pie.

Cereals. Cooked cereal, unsweetened muesli, and bran

flakes are slow to release sugar into the bloodstream, which helps raise serotonin levels.

Cottage cheese. It's high in tryptophan, which is lacking in people with SAD. Other foods just as high in tryptophan are turkey, fish, and eggs.

Ice. When you can't get going no matter what you do, try sucking on some ice. Its chill can give you a wake-up call. Or, splash your face and wrists with ice water.

Legumes. Eating these can help maintain an even serotonin level throughout the day and night.

Shellfish. These are high in tyrosine, which forms chemicals that act on the brain cells to improve concentration and alertness, both of which become sluggish with SAD. Other foods high in tyrosine are fish, chicken, skinless turkey, cottage cheese, plain yogurt, skim milk, eggs, tofu, and very lean ham, pork, and lamb.

Turkey. Protein foods such as turkey, low fat cottage cheese, chicken, and low fat dairy products can reduce the carbohydrate cravings of SAD as well as control the weight gain that occurs during SAD months.

Herbal Remedies

Herbal teas. Any herbal tea is a better choice than teas with caffeine. Your reduced energy level may cause you to turn to caffeine for a boost, but it can also cause anxiety, muscle tension, and stomach problems, so opt for herbal. Chamomile, peppermint, and cinnamon are pleasant-tasting choices. Drink a cup instead of giving in to your carbohydrate cravings.

Peppermint oil. Or lemon oil. Steep in water and inhale. These are stimulating and may give you a little extra zip.

Stress

Stress. We all know what that's about, don't we? The traffic in your life is jamming up. Everything is fast-paced, high-pressured, loaded with responsibility. Some people thrive on that roller-coaster rhythm, but others don't, and the stresses in their lives begin to take a toll, physically and mentally. Stress alters body chemistry and affects immunity.

You know that heart attack someone suffered because he was "all stressed out"? Stress changed his body chemistry; it contributed to a hormonal imbalance that increased the rate at which plaque was hardening his arteries, and it altered the production and distribution of his body fat. The result of his stress: heart attack. And that psoriasis she suffers? Stress caused her nerve cells to produce a chemical that stopped immune cells from fighting the red, itchy skin disease she's plagued with.

Dietary Remedies

Celery. The phytonutrients called phthalides found in celery have a widely recognized sedative effect, so eat your celery raw or chopped into a salad.

Cherries. They soothe the nervous system and relieve stress. Eat them fresh or any way you like them.

Lettuce. This stress-reducing veggie has a sedative effect. A small amount of lacturcarium, a natural sedative, is found in the white, milky juice that oozes from the lettuce when the stalk is snapped.

Oats. Besides fighting off high cholesterol, oats produce a calming effect that fights off stress. Use them in bread recipes and desserts or for thickening in soups. Or just eat a bowl of oatmeal!

Pasta. When you're faced with eating a late-night meal, choose pasta. It causes a rise in the brain chemical serotonin, which has a calming effect on the body. Rice produces the same effect.

Whole-wheat bread. It's high in the B vitamins, which sustain the nervous system. Other B-rich foods include whole-wheat pita bread, whole-grain cereal, pasta, and brown rice. For a good stress-fighting diet, about 60 percent of your daily calories should come from these starchy foods, divided among your meals.

Herbal Remedies

Cardamom seeds. These are said to freshen the breath, speed the digestion, and cheer the heart, and they also bust the stress. To make a tea, cover 2 to 3 pods with boiling water and steep for ten minutes. Cardamom pods can be added to a regular pot of tea, too, in order to derive the calming effect. Also, crush the pods and add to rice or lentils before cooking, or use in a vegetable stir-fry. If you like the taste, cardamom seeds are a good addition to cakes and biscuits. Instead of pods, you can use 1 teaspoon powdered cardamom, which is available in the spice section of the grocery store.

Peppermint. Drink a cup of peppermint tea before bed to relieve tension and help you sleep. Chamomile, catnip, or vervain works well, too. Place 1 teaspoon of the dried leaf in a cup of boiling water. Sweeten with honey and sip before bed. To reap the fullest benefits, sipping this soothing tea should be the last thing you do before you tuck yourself in for the night. During the day, if you don't have time for a cup of tea, try a peppermint. Read the label for a good variety, though. One with peppermint, sugar, and little else is best. The more extra ingredients that go into the candy, the less the relaxing benefit.

Tarragon. A tarragon tea calms the nervous system. Add 1/2 teaspoon dried tarragon to 1 cup boiling water. Or use it fresh, snipped into salads or vegetables. It's a good seasoning for creamy soups, too, or added to a salad dressing of balsamic vinegar with a dash of honey.

Topical Remedies

Baking soda. A soothing bath in baking soda and ginger can relieve stress. Add 1/3 cup ginger and 1/3 cup baking soda to a tub of hot water and enjoy the soak.

Salt. Try this muscle-soothing bath to wash that stress away. Mix 1/2 cup salt, 1 cup Epsom salts, and 2 cups baking soda. Add 1/2 cup of the mix to your bathwater. Store the dry mix in a covered container, away from moisture.

Sesame oil. For a nice relaxation technique, warm a few ounces and rub it all over your body, from head to toe. Sunflower and corn oil work well, too. After your massage, take a long, hot soak in the tub.

Teething

Your baby's first tooth is certainly a time for rejoicing. It's a real milestone in her life. And it also explains why your kid has been a drool factory, why she's been sticking anything and everything into her mouth lately, and why she's been so cranky. By the time that first tooth cuts through the gums, your

baby has endured swollen, painful, inflamed gums for days or even
months. They don't call it "cutting"
teeth for nothing. Getting those
first teeth is an ordeal for any kid.

Babies actually have tooth buds
in place, resting right under the
gums, before they're born. Those
teeth then push their way through
the gums, making their debut anywhere from four to eight months
of age. The process of getting primary teeth continues until close to
the third birthday. Your sweet pea
will probably get her bottom front
teeth first, followed by her top front
teeth. Don't fret if she has huge
gaps between teeth or if the teeth
grow in a little crooked. Things
will straighten out over time. By
the time your little one is finished
getting that first set of teeth, she'll
have 20 munching, crunching teeth.
These will stay in place until she's
ready for permanent teeth, sometime around her sixth birthday.

Teething is, of course, just a
part of life. But there are some
things you can grab at home that
will ease your baby's discomfort
and make her a happy camper.

Dietary Remedies

Applesauce. Cold foods like
straight-from-the-fridge applesauce
taste good and are gum-friendly.

Topical Remedies

Baby bottle. One trick for making baby happier during teething is
to put water in a baby bottle and
freeze the bottle upside down (so
the water is frozen at the nipple).
Give it to the baby when he gets
fussy and let him chew on the cold,
comforting nipple for a while.

Bagels. Refrigerate an ordinary
bagel and it becomes your very
own homemade teething ring. It's
great for babies to gum on while
they're getting teeth in and can
help ease that teething ache.

Bananas. Stick a banana in the
freezer and then let baby put the
soothing, sweet treat to her gums.

Carrots. Get a carrot out of
the fridge, wash it thoroughly or peel it, and let your baby
gum it to her heart's content.

Dishcloth. Put a clean wet dishcloth or towel in the refrigerator

and let it get nice and cold. Then give it to junior and let him gnaw away on the cloth. This will help ease inflamed gums and will feel good in baby's mouth.

Ice. Wrap some ice in a dishtowel and let baby suck on the towel. The cold ice will keep swelling down and ease baby's pain. But don't let her suck on just the ice as it can harm your baby's gums.

Spoon. Take a tip from the American Dental Association, stick a spoon in the fridge for a few hours and then let baby have at it. The cold metal against her gums will put a smile on her face.

Teething biscuit. These hard, unsweetened, crackerlike biscuits are great for gnawing on when teeth are making their way through the gums.

Ulcers

An ulcer is a sore or hole in the protective mucosal lining of the gastrointestinal tract. Ulcers appear in the area of the stomach or the duodenum, the upper part of the small intestine, where caustic digestive juices, pepsin, and hydrochloric acid are present. Today we know

that the majority of ulcers are the result of an infection with a bacteria called *Helicobacter pylori* (*H. pylori*). This bacteria makes the stomach and small intestine more susceptible to the erosive effects of the digestive juices. The bacteria may also cause the stomach to produce more acid.

There are some lifestyle factors that can contribute to the development of an ulcer. These include alcohol consumption, eating and drinking foods that contain caffeine, significant physical (not emotional) stress such as severe burns and major surgery, and excessive use of certain over-the-counter pain medications such as aspirin or ibuprofen. Studies have shown that smoking also tends to increase the chances of developing an ulcer, slows the healing of existing ulcers, and makes a recurrence more likely. Family history of ulcers also appears to play a role in susceptibility.

Researchers believe some people just produce more stomach acid than others. If stomach acid production isn't the problem, then a weak stomach may be. The stomach lining in certain individuals may be less able to withstand the onslaught of gastric acids. Lifestyle factors mentioned above can also weaken the stomach's lining.

You're probably familiar with the most typical symptom of a brewing ulcer: a burning or gnawing pain between the breastbone and navel. This pain is more common between meals (it improves with eating but returns a few hours later) and in the middle of the night or toward dawn. Less typical symptoms include nausea or vomiting, weight loss and loss of appetite, and frequent burping or bloating.

If you have an ulcer or suspect you may have one, you should be under the care of a physician. Between visits to the doctor, there are ways to care for your digestive tract.

Dietary Remedies

Bananas. These fruits contain an antibacterial substance that may inhibit the growth of ulcer-causing *H. pylori*. And studies show that animals fed bananas have a thicker stomach wall and greater mucus production in the stomach, which helps build a better barrier between digestive acids and the lining of the stomach. Eating plantains is also helpful.

Cabbage. Researchers have found that ulcer patients who drink 1 quart of raw cabbage juice per day can often heal their ulcers in five days. If chugging a quart of cabbage juice turns your stomach inside out, researchers also found that those who eat plain cabbage have quicker healing times as well. Time for some coleslaw!

Garlic. Garlic's antibacterial properties include fighting *H. pylori*. Take two small crushed cloves per day.

Plums. Red- and purple-colored foods inhibit the growth of *H. pylori*. Like plums, berries can help you fight the good fight, too.

Herbal Remedies

Cayenne pepper. Used moderately, a little cayenne pepper can go a long way in helping ulcers. The pepper stimulates blood flow to bring nutrients to the stomach. To make a cup of peppered tea, mix 1/4 teaspoon cayenne pepper in 1 cup hot water. Drink a cup per day. A dash of cayenne pepper can also be added to soups, meats, and other savory dishes.

Licorice. Several modern studies have demonstrated the ulcer-healing abilities of licorice. Licorice does its part not by reducing stomach acid but rather by reducing the ability of stomach acid to damage stomach lining. Properties in licorice encourage digestive mucosal tissues to protect themselves from acid. Licorice can be used in encapsulated form, but for a quick cup of licorice tea, cut 1 ounce licorice root into slices and cover with 1 quart boiling water. Steep, cool, and strain. (If licorice root is unavailable, cut 1 ounce licorice sticks into slices.) You can also try licorice candy if it's made with real licorice (the label will say "licorice mass") and not just flavored with anise. Don't eat more than 1 ounce per day.

Urinary Tract Infection

Urinary tract infections (UTIs) are the second most common reason people visit their doctors each year. Men get UTIs, but they are much more common in women. More than eight million women head to their doctor for UTI treatment annually. And 20 percent of these women will get a second UTI.

If you've ever had a UTI, you'll probably never forget the symptoms. It usually starts with a sudden and frequent need to visit the restroom. When you get there, you can squeeze out only a little bit of urine, and that's usually accompanied by a burning sensation in your bladder and/or urethra. In more extreme cases, you may end up with fever, chills, back pain, and even blood in your urine.

UTIs are a result of bacteria, particularly *Escherichia coli* (*E. coli*) bacteria, taking temporary control of your bladder and your urethra (the tube that allows urine to flow from your bladder to the toilet). Women tend to get more UTIs for two reasons: They have a shorter urethra than men, and their urethral opening is precariously close to the vagina and the anus, where *E. coli* and other bacteria normally hang out without causing harm. That means everyday body functions and sex are more likely to push bacteria into your urethra. Being pregnant also ups your risk of a UTI because your bladder is under a lot of pressure from your uterus and is more apt to entertain an infection. And if you use a diaphragm to protect against pregnancy, you put more pressure on your urethra and are more likely to end up with a UTI.

Men get UTIs but not for the same reasons. If a man suspects he has a UTI, he should call his doctor;

the UTI may be due to a bladder stone, an enlarged prostate, or a sexually transmitted disease such as gonorrhea. A prostate infection may also make its way to the bladder, causing a bladder infection.

UTIs that last longer than two days require medical intervention. Untreated UTIs can infect the kidneys and turn into a much more serious problem. To help prevent a UTI from developing or nip one in the bud, try some of the remedies available in your own home.

Dietary Remedies

Baking soda. Adding 1 teaspoon baking soda to your glass of water may help ease your infection. The soda neutralizes the acidity in your urine, speeding along your recovery.

Blueberries. Blueberries and cranberries are from the same plant family and seem to have the same bacteria-inhibiting properties. In one study, blueberry juice was found to prevent UTIs. Since you're not likely to find a gallon of blueberry juice at your local store, try sprinkling a handful of these flavorful, good-for-you berries over your morning cereal.

Cranberry juice. Many studies have found that drinking cranberry juice may help you avoid urinary tract infections. It appears that cranberry juice prevents infection-causing bacteria from bedding down in your bladder, and it also has a very mild antibiotic affect. Drinking as little as 4 ounces of cranberry juice per day can help keep your bladder infection-free. If you tend to get UTIs or are dealing with one right now, try to drink at least 2 to 4 glasses of cranberry juice per day. If pure cranberry juice is just too bitter for your taste buds, you can substitute cranberry juice cocktail. It seems to have the same effect as the pure stuff. Take note: If you have a UTI, cranberry juice is not a replacement for doctor-prescribed antibiotics in treating your infection.

Pineapple. Bromelain is an enzyme found in pineapples. In one study, people with a UTI who were given bromelain along with their usual round of antibiotics got rid of their infection. Only half the people who were given a placebo plus an antibiotic showed no signs of lingering infection. Eating a cup of pineapple tastes good and may just help rid you of your infection.

Water. If you tend to get urinary tract infections, be sure to drink plenty of water, about 8 eight-ounce glasses a day. You should be urinating at least every four to five hours. If you are currently dealing with an infection, drink buckets of water to fight it off. Drink a full 8 ounces of water every hour. The river of water in your system will help flush out bacteria by making you urinate more frequently.

Dietary Supplement Remedies

Vitamin C. Some doctors are prescribing at least 5,000 mg or more of vitamin C per day for patients who develop recurrent urinary tract infections. Vitamin C keeps the bladder healthy by acidifying the urine, essentially putting up a no-trespassing sign for potentially harmful bacteria.

Herbal Remedies

Goldenseal. This herb is a well-known infection fighter. It has a component called berberine that works much like cranberry juice in keeping harmful bacteria from camping out in your bladder. The typical recommended dose is 250 to 400 mg of goldenseal root extract containing 10 percent berberine, three times per day.

Uva ursi. European doctors prescribe this herb for urinary tract infections. This herb has a chemical that is converted by your urine to a bacteria-killing machine. If you have a urinary tract infection, the recommended amount of this herb is 3 to 5 mL of an uva ursi tincture three times per day.

Topical Remedies

Hot water. Heat up some water on the stove, and pour it into a hot water bottle. Place the water bottle on your lower abdomen to help ease any pain caused by the infection.

Warts

Warts are caused by the human papillomavirus (HPV), and there are more than 60 varieties of it. You get a wart from coming into contact with the virus through skin-to-skin contact. You can get the virus from another person, via a handshake for example, or you can actually give one to yourself if you already have a wart. You can spread the wart virus to other parts of your body by scratching, touching, shaving, or even biting your nails. All it takes is a little break in the skin for the virus to enter the system.

Before you can attempt to get rid of your wart, you have to be sure that little bump actually is one. There are three common varieties: common, plantar, and flat, according to the American Academy of Dermatology.

Common warts are found in areas where the skin has been broken: where fingernails are bitten down to the quick or hangnails are picked until they bleed. Often, they look like they have little dots or seeds in them, which is why they're frequently called "seed warts." But what you see aren't seeds; they're merely dots produced by the blood vessel supplying the infected area.

Plantar warts do not stick above the surface the way common warts do. That's because the pressure from walking pushes them back into the skin.

Flat warts are the smallest of the warts. These warts are found in clumps of 20 to 100, usually on the face and neck, but also on the chest, knees, hands, wrists, and forearms. In men, they're common in the bearded area, most likely picked up from shaving irritations and nicks. In women, they're common on shaved legs.

There are many ways to rid yourself of a wart. Doctors can zap them with a laser, burn or freeze them, or give you topical medications that might do the trick. However, there might just be a home remedy that will send your unsightly little nuisance into wart oblivion.

Dietary Remedies

Foods. Eat foods that strengthen the immune system, such as broccoli, garlic, oranges, onions, red meats, rice, scallions, sunflower seeds, sweet potatoes, whole-grain breads.

Dietary Supplement Remedies

Vitamin C. Crush 1 vitamin C tablet, and add water to make a thick paste. Apply it to the wart, then cover. The acid in the vitamin C may irritate the wart away.

Vitamin E. Break a vitamin E or A capsule, rub a little of the oil on the wart, and cover it with an adhesive bandage. Repeat three times per day. Remove the bandage at night to let it breathe, then start over with the oil in the morning.

Topical Remedies

Adhesive tape. Wrap a finger wart with four layers of adhesive tape. Wrap the first strip over the top of the finger and the second strip around the finger. Repeat both wrappings. Leave the adhesive in place 6 1/2 days, then remove and let the wart breathe for half a day. Repeat the process until the wart is gone.

Baking powder. Mix baking powder and castor oil into a paste, then apply it to the wart at night, covering it with a bandage. Remove bandage the next morning. Repeat as necessary.

Baking soda. Dissolve baking soda in water, then wash your wart-plagued hand or foot in it. Let your hand dry naturally, with the baking soda still on it. Repeat often, until the wart is gone.

Carrots. Finely grate a carrot and add enough olive oil to it to make a paste. Dab the paste on your wart twice daily for 30 minutes for two to three weeks.

Figs. Mash up a fresh fig and place some on your wart for 30 minutes. Do this daily for two to three weeks.

Lemon juice. Squeeze a little lemon juice on your wart, then cover it with fresh, chopped onions for 30 minutes once per day for two to three weeks.

Pineapple juice. Soak your wart in pineapple juice. It has a dissolving enzyme.

Herbal Remedies

Aloe. Break open an aloe leaf, and soak up the clear juice from the inner leaf on a cotton ball. Apply the cotton ball to the wart, and cover with a bandage. Repeat daily until the wart is gone.

Garlic. Rub crushed garlic or onion on your wart. Or eat fresh garlic. If you don't want to smell like an Italian cookery, try swallowing three garlic capsules three times per day, or munch on some breath-freshening parsley afterward.

More Do's & Don'ts

- 🐾 Don't scratch existing warts.
- 🐾 Don't shake hands with someone who has an obvious wart.
- 🐾 Use an electric razor if the area you shave has a wart.
- 🐾 Wash your hands with soap and hot water if you've touched a wart.
- 🐾 Keep it dry. Warts love to multiply in moist areas.

Water Retention

Water retention is part of the premenstrual syndrome (PMS) package. During this time, hormonal fluctuations can cause havoc in a woman's body. In some women, the monthly rise in estrogen turns on the faucet for the hormone aldosterone. Aldosterone, in turn, causes the kidneys to retain fluids and the woman to suddenly gain a few water-filled pounds.

Although PMS is the major cause of water retention in women, water retention for both men and women can also be related to kidney problems, both serious (kidney disease) and commonplace (not drinking enough water). Heart, liver, or thyroid malfunctions can also play a role in water retention. And, of course, eating too many salty foods can turn your body into a water-storage tank.

Thanks to the effects of gravity, retained water tends to flow southward and pool in the feet, ankles, and legs, although no area of the body is immune. Try to elevate your legs frequently. If you suffer from the occasional bloated-cow feeling due to PMS, eating too much, or not drinking enough water, there are ways to deflate yourself at home.

Dietary Remedies

Bananas. Go ape and grab a few bananas. Slice 'em on your cereal, make a smoothie, or just peel and eat them plain. Bananas contain high amounts of potassium, which helps eliminate fluid retention. Not a banana fan? Gobble down a handful of raisins instead.

Cabbage. A natural diuretic, cabbage can be added to salads or sandwiches. Enjoy a side of coleslaw for lunch.

Cranberry juice. Another natural diuretic. Drink it straight from the bottle.

Salt. Around the time you expect your period, drastically reduce your salt intake. Sodium increases fluid retention, so don't use the salt shaker. If recipes call for salt, try adding more pepper or another spice instead. Most importantly, cut down on processed foods and fast foods, all of which are overflowing with salt.

Water. When you feel water-logged, guzzling a glass of H2O might be the last thing on your mind, but it may be the best thing for you. Water flushes out the system better than anything else and can reduce premenstrual bloating. Drink 8 to 10 glasses per day; more when you exercise.

Yogurt. Too many rich treats will cause stomachs to bloat. If you've overindulged and are feeling the effects, treat your stomach to a cup of plain, low fat yogurt that contains active cultures. The active cultures aid in digestion and increase the good bacteria in the gut.

Dietary Supplement Remedies

Vitamins A and C. When you feel like a balloon, try to increase your intake of vitamins A and C, both of which help diminish the fragility of capillaries and decrease water retention.

Topical Remedies

Ice. When ankles puff up, applying an ice pack can help bring them back to normal size. Place ice cubes in a plastic bag with a zipper seal, wrap a light towel around the bag, and apply for five to ten minutes. A bag of frozen veggies also works well. In summertime, dip legs (ankle-deep) into a bath of ice water. People who have diabetes or poor circulation in their feet should skip the ice bath, however, unless directed to use it by their physician.

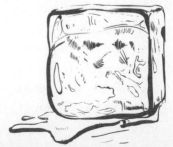

Yeast Infection

No one wants to talk about a yeast infection, and no one wants to admit they have one. That's probably because it's known as one of those "personal" things that only affects women. Well, in most cases that's true, but yeast infections are not restricted to women only. You know that diaper rash covering the cutest little bottom you've ever seen? Guess what? Yeast. And that condition called thrush that babies often develop in the mouth? Yeast again. So you see, yeast is not just about an unpleasant vaginal infection that no one wants to talk about.

Yeast happens when the acidity of normal fluids is altered. Usually they're acidic enough to keep the yeast from flourishing. But when something goes wrong, the balance is tipped and the yeast have a party, multiplying over and over.

Yeast infections also can be transmitted between sexual partners. Using condoms or abstaining from sex during the infection are the best ways to prevent spreading it. Typical symptoms of a vaginal yeast infection include intense itching and soreness accompanied by a thick white discharge. Symptoms of a genital yeast infection in men include irritation and itching in the genital area, sometimes accompanied by white discharge under the foreskin and/or swelling at the end of the penis. In the throat, yeast looks like creamy white patches.

Most yeast infections can be cured with remedies found on the pharmacy shelf either in cream or suppository form. There are also prescription medications available that will stop the problem in as little as three days. The following are some simple home panaceas that can bring relief or cure and even stop the disease from recurring.

Dietary Remedies

Cranberry juice. Drink this one. Unsweetened, it may acidify vaginal secretions and equip them to fight off the yeast.

Yogurt. The live culture in plain yogurt is a great remedy for a yeast infection, helping to restore the acid-bacteria balance in more ways than one. Of course, you can eat yogurt. You can also insert 1 to 2 tablespoons into your vagina, apply it externally to the affected area (anal or vaginal), or use it as a douche by diluting it with warm water.

Salt. If mouth sores develop with thrush, gargle with a mixture of 1/2 cup lukewarm water and 1/2 teaspoon salt to promote healing.

Water. For a baby with thrush, give 1/2 ounce boiled, cooled water after a feeding to wash away milk remnants that contain milk sugars, which yeast love to feed on.

Herbal Remedies

Basil. For thrush, make a basil tea and use it as a gargle. Boil 3 1/2 cups water, remove from heat, and add 1 1/4 teaspoons ground basil. Cover and steep for 30 minutes. Cool and gargle. Or sweeten to taste with maple syrup and drink 1 cup twice per day.

Garlic. Eating 2 fresh garlic cloves a day, either plain or minced and tossed in a salad or sauce, may prevent yeast infections or help clear up a case of thrush. Garlic has antifungal properties.

Rosemary. To relieve itching and burning, make a tea of rosemary, and use it as a douche or dab it onto the external area.

Thyme. Make a thyme tea using 1 teaspoon dried thyme per 1 cup boiling water. Steep and drink 1 to 4 cups per day if you have a yeast infection.

Topical Remedies

Baking soda. For thrush, brush your teeth after every meal with a mild toothpaste of baking soda and water. Commercial toothpaste may be too harsh if sores develop. Pour a little baking soda in your hand and add just enough water to make a paste. Then, rinse with 1/2 cup warm water and 1 tablespoon of three percent hydrogen peroxide. Replace your toothbrush when the infection is cured.

Licorice powder. Boil 1 pint water and add 1 teaspoon licorice powder. Steep it, strain, but don't drink. Use the liquid as a vaginal douche.

Vinegar. Make a mild vinegar douche and use at the first sign of problems. Mix 1 to 3 tablespoons white vinegar with 1 quart of water.